NERVE AND MUSCLE E

NERVE *and* MUSCLE EXCITATION

EXCITATION

THIRD EDITION

Douglas Junge

UNIVERSITY OF CALIFORNIA
LOS ANGELES

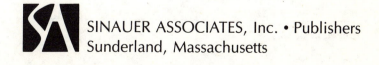

SINAUER ASSOCIATES, Inc. • Publishers
Sunderland, Massachusetts

NERVE AND MUSCLE EXCITATION, Third Edition

Library of Congress Cataloging-in-Publication Data

Junge, Douglas.
    Nerve and muscle excitation / Douglas Junge. — 3rd ed.
       p.   cm.
    Includes bibliographical references and index.
    ISBN 0-87893-406-5 (paper)
    1. Action potentials (Electrophysiology) 2. Nerves. 3. Muscles.
4. Excitation (Physiology)   I. Title.
   [DNLM: 1. Action Potentials. WL 102 J95n]
QP341.J86 1992
591.1′88—dc20
DNLM/DLC
for Library of Congress   91-4994
                                      CIP

Printed in U.S.A.

5 4 3 2 1

For Janice

CONTENTS

PREFACE

In attempting to understand the functions of nervous systems, scientists have followed a reductionist path: To analyze a process such as inhibition of activity in one part of a nervous system by excitation in another, one needs to study the electrical activity of the single nerve cells involved. Some results of this work may be that the cell membrane potentials become more negative during a volley of activity in an inhibitory nerve, and more positive during an excitatory input. These positive changes may cause action potentials in some of the postsynaptic cells, and the inhibitory input may make it more difficult for them to excite these cells. So far, so good: Excitation is a positive change in membrane potential; inhibition is (sometimes) a negative change, and the study has produced a new level of understanding.

But new quandaries emerge: What is the mechanism of the excitation? Is it chemical or electrical in nature? And how does one nerve excite another, or a muscle, or a gland cell? More basic studies are required with different ionic solutions, and drugs that block specific currents. After a time we know that during nerve excitation sodium carries the inward current and potassium the outward, and that during muscle excitation the postsynaptic membrane becomes permeable to many different cations.

Still, we might inquire: How do those charged bits of matter traverse the nerve or muscle (or gland) membrane? Are there "ferry boats" that pick up a sodium ion on the outside and a potassium on the inside, and carry them both to the opposite sides? Or do little "pores" open, letting a certain amount of ions flow down their concentration gradients? In the laboratory, with higher-gain amplifiers and lower-noise electrodes, we find smaller things to examine, such as gating currents and single-channel currents. We discover that membrane currents are made up of microscopic quantized currents flowing through channels that open and close under the influence of membrane potential and external chemical transmitters. This is the study of biological processes at the single-molecule (channel) level.

Now, the possibility arises of asking a fundamental question: What genes determine the formation of what channels? It is just such a lack of these genes--and the consequent missing channel--that results in a disease such as muscular dystrophy. Although the process of reductionism may be extended to the atomic nucleus one day, for now molecular neurobiology promises to occupy at least a generation of biophysicists.

This book has been revised to include some of the breathtaking developments in the field during the past decade. It was clear during the reworking process that much of the earlier work with excitable membranes has stood up well and should be examined by students of nerves and muscles. Other subjects did not seem central in retrospect and have been abandoned. Many topics have not been included due to the sheer volume of research in cellular neurophysiology. If any unifying theme has been chosen, it is the availability of theoretical models in a given topic area.

The author is indebted to Elba E. Serrano and Malcolm Brodwick for reading individual sections, and to Gregory Lnenicka, Andrew Harris, and Bruce Johnson for valuable suggestions about the revision. He especially thanks Daniel Kalman for comments on the overall manuscript.

Los Angeles
March 1, 1991

IMPORTANT QUANTITIES
USED IN THIS BOOK

CONSTANTS

R =	universal gas constant	= 8.3144 joules/kg · mol · degree
F =	Faraday constant	= 96,500 coulombs/mol charge
e =	natural base	= 2.71828
N_o =	Avogadro's number	= 6.023×10^{23} molecules/mole

UNITS

Å =	angstrom (unit of length)	= 10^{-8} cm
A =	ampere (unit of current)	= 1 coulomb/sec
Da =	dalton (unit of mol wt)	= 1 g/mol
F =	farad (unit of capacitance)	= 1 coulomb/volt
J =	joule (unit of work)	= 1 volt · coulomb
S =	siemen (unit of conductance)	= 1 ampere/volt

VARIABLES

T = temperature, Kelvin   = temperature, °C + 273

$$\text{erf } x = \text{error function} \qquad = \frac{2}{\sqrt{\pi}} \int_0^x e^{-x^2}\, dx$$

$$\ln x = \text{natural logarithm} \qquad = \frac{\log x}{\log e} = 2.3026 \log x$$

But man does not limit himself to seeing; he thinks and insists on learning the meaning of the phenomena whose existence has been revealed to him by observation. So he reasons, compares facts, puts questions to them, and by the answers which he extracts, tests one by another.

Claude Bernard, 1865
An Introduction to the Study of Experimental Medicine

1

ELECTRICAL RECORDINGS FROM NEURONS AND SINGLE MUSCLE FIBERS

Extracellular stimulation and recording techniques were among the first to be used in electrophysiology, and they are still actively employed. Therefore, a brief consideration of these methods is relevant to the study of excitable membranes. A typical arrangement for extracellular studies with an isolated section of nerve is shown in Figure 1. The nerve is laid over a row of silver wires in a hermetically sealed moist chamber with a small amount of saline on the bottom. This method produces much larger signals than recording under the saline solution, as it avoids shunting of the recorded signals. A pair of wires at one end of the nerve is connected to a stimulator (S) that produces short voltage pulses to excite the nerve. A pair at the other end is connected to a differential high-gain ac preamplifier (A) that prepares the signal for display on the oscilloscope (OS). The preamplifier must be differential, that is have (+) and (−) inputs, because the nerve signals to be recorded are usually the same size or smaller than the 60-Hz interference in each lead. By subtracting the signal at the (+) lead from that at the (−) lead one can minimize this interference. The gain must be high, as the extracellular signals are typically in the microvolt range. The preamplifier must also have a high input impedance, or it will shunt the signals and reduce the amplitude. Typical input impedances for biological preamplifiers of this sort are greater than 100 MΩ.

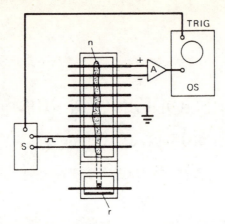

1

Experimental arrangement for extracellular recording of nerve action potentials. n, nerve; r, Ringer's solution in bottom of chamber; TRIG, trigger signal.

THE COMPOUND ACTION POTENTIAL

The sequence of events during stimulation of the nerve and display of the extracellular action potential is: (1) The stimulator emits a brief trigger pulse that starts the oscilloscope beam moving horizontally across the screen. (2) After a certain delay, the stimulator emits a square stimulus pulse (may be 0.1 to 2.0 msec, 1 to 10V). As the amplitude of the pulse is increased, it excites some of the axons that make up the piece of nerve. (3) The action potential generated is picked up by the recording electrode pair and produces a trace on the oscilloscope such as that shown on the left of Figure 2. This is called a COMPOUND ACTION POTENTIAL because it is made up of the summed activity of hundreds of axons. We can understand the shape of this action potential by considering the activity of a single axon, as shown in Figure 2, right. The resting distribution of charges across the axon membrane is negative inside, as shown on the left of the drawings. At time 1 the nerve impulse, consisting of a region of reversed polarity (positive inside), reaches the first external recording electrode. This causes the negative deflection in the voltage trace seen at the top of the figure. At time 2 the impulse has moved along the axon to a point halfway between the recording electrodes, so the recorded potential returns to zero. At time 3 the impulse has reached the second electrode, and a positive deflection is seen. This entire event is usually referred to as a BIPHASIC ACTION POTENTIAL. The compound action potential recorded outside the whole nerve (left) results from hundreds of such

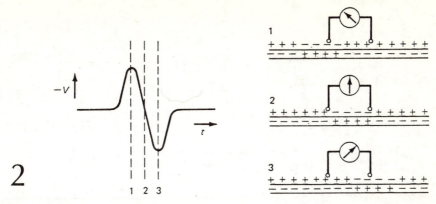

2

Biphasic action potential. Left: Shape of the extracellular potential when many axons in a nerve are excited synchronously. Right: Explanation of biphasic potential in terms of activity of a single nerve fiber.

miniature spikes occurring almost synchronously. The individual axon spikes are ALL-OR-NONE, that is, they will occur in exactly the same stereotyped way each time the stimulus exceeds the THRESHOLD level (which varies from axon to axon). The compound action potential, on the other hand, is GRADED and varies in size with the stimulus amplitude. This is because increasing the stimulus brings more and more axons into play, each of which contributes to the total record.

In another method of extracellular recording, one recording electrode is placed on a crushed end of the nerve, which is therefore unable to conduct. This produces a constant INJURY CURRENT between the recording electrodes because the crushed end is negative with respect to the uninjured portion. However, this current is usually not recorded by the ac preamplifiers used for extracellular recording. As the impulse passes down the nerve, an action potential such as that in Figure 3, left, is recorded. The entire event has a negative polarity because the positive phase has been removed by crushing the nerve under one electrode. This can be understood if we consider the behavior of one of the axons in the nerve, as shown on the right of the figure. The recorded signal is always negative as the impulse (1) approaches, (2) encounters, and (3) passes the active recording electrode. Because the crushed end is inactive, the impulse cannot pass by it and reverse the direction of current flow between the electrodes as in Figure 2. This technique is often called KILLED-END RECORDING, and the action potentials recorded by this method are called MONOPHASIC.

Nerve membranes also have the property of REFRACTORINESS fol-

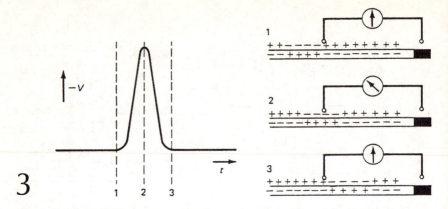

Monophasic action potential obtained with killed-end recording. Left: Extra-cellular potential recorded from many axons. Right: Explanation based on activity of a single fiber.

lowing an action potential: For a short time (less than 1 msec) follow-ing a spike in a single axon, no second action potential can be elicited, even if the stimulus is greatly increased. This is known as the ABSO-LUTE REFRACTORY PERIOD. At a slightly longer time after the first action potential, a second one can be produced if the stimulus is made larger than that needed to elicit the first spike. This is the RELATIVE REFRAC-TORY PERIOD. In whole nerves, the refractoriness of single axons is seen in the following way: As two stimuli occur closer and closer together in time, more and more single axons become refractory, and the second compound action potential is gradually reduced to zero.

THE FROG NERVE

So far we have considered the activity of only a single group of axons in the nerve, all of which have about the same conduction velocity; thus, the individual axonal action potentials were conducted from the stimulating site to the recording site at about the same rate and could sum to give distinct compound action potentials. However, almost all peripheral nerves have more than one group of fibers with particular conduction velocities. For example, in the frog peroneal nerve at least three different peaks can be resolved in the compound action potential (Figure 4) obtained with killed-end recording. As the stimulus ampli-tude is increased, the first peak to appear is that labeled α. As the stimulus amplitude is further increased, first the β and then the γ

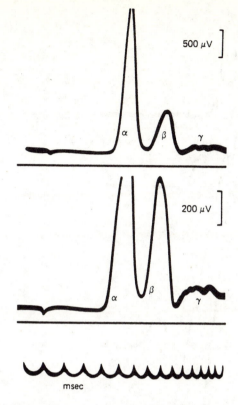

500 μV

200 μV

4

msec

Compound action potential from frog peroneal nerve, obtained with killed-end recording. α, β, and γ peaks due to different conduction velocities of groups of axons in the nerve. (Time scale compressed on right.) (From Erlanger and Gasser, 1937.)

deflections appear. This is because the fibers giving rise to the α peak have the lowest threshold. They also have the largest conduction velocity, as the α peak occurs earliest after the stimulus artifact (small downward deflection). This illustrates the general rule-of-thumb that fibers with the lowest threshold have the greatest conduction velocity.

Figure 5 shows Erlanger and Gasser's demonstration that the α and β peaks represent the activity of groups of fibers having different conduction velocities. Killed-end recording was used at one end of the nerve, and closely spaced pairs of stimulating electrodes were placed at various distances from the crushed end, indicated on the left margin. When the stimulating pair was very close to the recording electrode (top trace), the α and β deflections overlapped. As the conduction

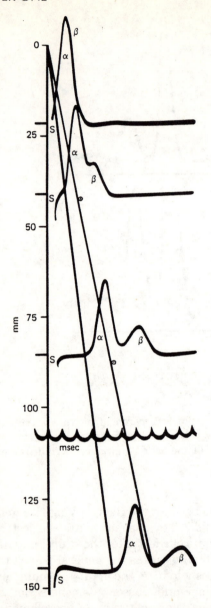

5

Demonstration that α and β peaks represent the activity of fiber groups with different conduction velocities. Numbers to left are distances in millimeters from stimulating electrode pair to recording electrode. (S indicates time of stimulus.) (From Erlanger and Gasser, 1937.)

distance was increased, the two deflections became more and more separated in time. This could only have been because the fiber groups giving rise to each deflection had different (but constant) conduction velocities. The slanting lines are drawn through the estimated beginning of the α and β deflection in each trace. The steeper slope of the α line indicates the greater conduction velocity of the α group of fibers.

VARIATION OF CONDUCTION VELOCITY WITH FIBER DIAMETER

From measurements on histological sections of nerves, it is possible to construct histograms of the diameters of the fibers present. Such a histogram for a human sensory nerve is shown in the inset of Figure 6. Two peaks are clearly present in the distribution of diameters; one has a mean of about 3 μm and the other has a mean of about 12 μm. The compound action potential for this nerve has the form shown in the graph of Figure 6, with two well-defined elevations. Erlanger and Gasser showed in several studies that the first, or fastest-conducted elevation was due to the large-diameter fiber group. They made hundreds of reconstructions of action potentials by making various assumptions about the contributions of individual fiber groups to the total record. The first, and most necessary assumption, was that the conduction velocity of each fiber was proportional to its outside diameter. By delaying the contribution of each size of fiber by the appropriate conduction time and summing, they could obtain a fair representation of the compound action potential. Erlanger and Gasser were able to obtain much better fits to the compound action potential assuming that individual spike amplitudes were proportional to fiber diameters. These assumptions were also found to hold for cat neurons (Hursh, 1939). A theoretical basis for the variation of spike amplitude and conduction velocity with fiber diameter will be given in the next chapter.

THE NODE OF RANVIER

The explanation of monophasic and biphasic action potentials in Figures 2 and 3 applies, strictly speaking, only to simple cylindrical axons. Real nerves almost always contain a large proportion of MYELINATED FIBERS. These have a multilayered coat of myelin membranes, longitudinally interrupted every 1 to 2 mm by a constriction called the NODE OF RANVIER. Here the insulating myelin disappears, and the central axon is exposed to the external solution, as diagrammed in Figure 7.

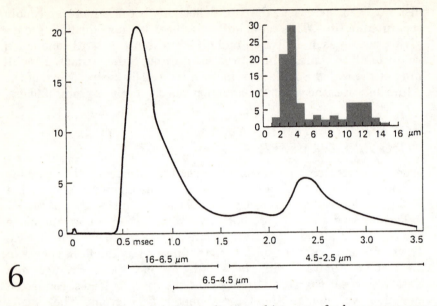

6

Compound action potential and fiber-diameter histogram for human sensory nerve. Ordinate scale in arbitrary units. Stimulus applied at time 0. Ranges of fiber diameters giving rise to each part of action potential indicated below. (From Gasser, 1943.)

Tasaki and Takeuchi (1941 and 1942) first showed that propagation of the nerve impulse in myelinated fibers occurs by SALTATORY CONDUCTION (from the Latin *saltare*, to dance). This process is illustrated in Figure 8, from the work of Huxley and Stämpfli (1949). The frog sciatic nerve was dissected down to a single myelinated fiber, and the fiber was pulled through an insulating barrier so that the potentials could be recorded from one side of the barrier to the other. The recorded potentials were proportional to the average longitudinal current inside the fiber between the two sides of the barrier. By taking the difference

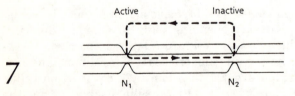

7

Myelinated nerve fiber, showing outward current at one node produced by activity in a neighboring node.

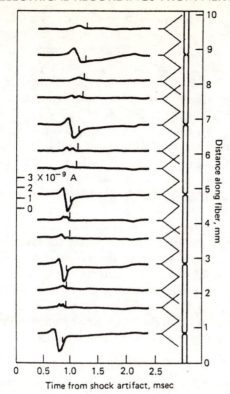

8

Saltatory conduction in myelinated fiber. Traces show currents recorded at various positions along the fiber. (From Huxley and Stämpfli, 1949.)

of the longitudinal currents at different regions of the fiber, Huxley and Stämpfli found the membrane current as a function of position along the fiber. (The Y shapes on the right indicate the position of the barrier at which the records were calculated.) Because the nerve was stimulated at the same position each time, the action currents occurred earlier and earlier as the barrier was moved along the fiber. It can be seen that only very small currents were recorded in the internodal regions, while large currents were recorded near the nodes. The action potential "hopped" from one node to the next. This is known to result from the excitation of an inactive node by activity in a neighboring node, as shown in Figure 7. The action potential at N_1 results from an inward flow of sodium ions (to be discussed in Chapters 3 and 5). This results in an outward flow of current at N_2, which excites the inactive node and produces an action potential there. About 0.1 msec after an action potential at one node, a new action potential suddenly appears at the next node, with no activity in the internodal region. This method of conduction contrasts with that in unmyelinated axons, where the action potential moves smoothly, without jumps.

In 1951, Huxley and Stämpfli came up with an ingenious method to measure the transmembrane potential of a single node, which is illustrated in Figure 9. The nodes N_1 and N_2 were insulated by two high-resistance gaps (g) in the external medium (one was filled with paraffin oil and the other was a thin layer of celluloid). Node N_1 was placed in normal Ringer's solution (an artificial solution similar to the extracellular body fluid), and node N_2 was placed in isotonic KCl, which depolarized it completely. One might think that the membrane resting potential could now be measured directly between N_1 and N_2, because N_1 had a normal resting potential E_r, and N_2 had none. However, even the small amount of saline under the gaps was enough to shunt, and greatly reduce, the measurable potential. Huxley and Stämpfli avoided this problem by measuring the short-circuit current flowing through the axoplasmic resistance (R) and under the insulating barriers in the path N_1N_2CBA. They measured this current as a voltage drop across the high barrier resistance from B to C. Then an external voltage V was applied between A and B and adjusted to re-

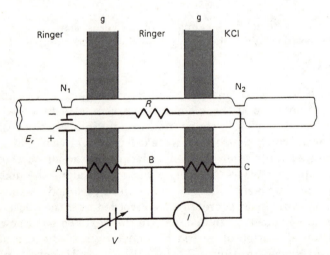

9

Potentiometric method of measuring transmembrane potentials in single node of Ranvier. V is adjusted until $I = 0$; then $V = -E_r$. (After Huxley and Stämpfli, 1951.)

duce the current to zero. This value of V was presumably equal and opposite to E_r, the potential giving rise to the short-circuit current. The average resting potential found by the investigators was -71 mV.

The method was even adapted to measurement of action-potential amplitudes; pulses of voltage that reduced the short-circuit current just to zero were applied from A to B at the peak of the action potential. The average value of overshoot measured in this way was $+45$ mV.

THE SUCROSE GAP

The successful recording of membrane potentials at the node of Ranvier led to the clever use of an extracellular insulating barrier for recording membrane potentials in whole axons or bundles of axons. In 1954, Stämpfli first described the method, and it was developed considerably by Julian et al. (1962a,b) using lobster axons. As shown in Figure 10, the insulating barriers are streams of sucrose flowing around the axon in such a way as to create three isolated sections of nerve. The two end sections are depolarized with KCl, and the central section is perfused with seawater, which is similar to the extracellular fluid, thus becoming an "artificial node." Membrane potentials can be measured from one KCl pool to the seawater pool, and currents may be injected via the other KCl pool. Stämpfli (1954) found that flowing sucrose was necessary to the success of this method, because petroleum jelly or another stationary insulator did not remove the ions adherent to the axons under the insulator. The sucrose gap method has been applied to many studies of nerve properties, especially with axons that are too small to impale with longitudinal electrodes, as described in the next section.

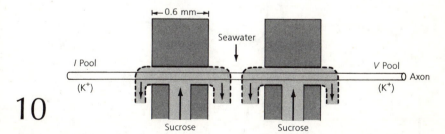

10

The sucrose gap method of measuring membrane potentials in axons. (From Julian et al., 1962a.)

INTRACELLULAR RECORDING

The development of the field was arrested for more than four years during World War II. In 1945, Hodgkin and Huxley were able to publish their studies, done in 1939, with direct intracellular measurements of resting and active membrane potentials in the squid giant axon. To make these observations, they had to use a high-impedance amplifier (10^{10} Ω) so as not to shunt the recorded signals. However, unlike with extracellular signals, the gain could be low, because the intracellular potentials were much larger (typically 50 to 100 mV). Also, the amplifier was a dc type, instead of the ac type used for extracellular measurements, so that they were able to amplify constant potential differences such as the resting potential. (These techniques were also used for dc measurements with the sucrose gap.)

The early capillary electrodes Hodgkin and Huxley used to record transmembrane potentials were about 100 μm in diameter and were introduced vertically into the cut end of a suspended length of axon. The glass capillary electrode was filled with seawater, and a silver wire ran inside along most of the length. One lead of the preamplifier was connected to the silver wire, and the other lead was connected to a coil of chlorided silver wire in the external solution. Stimuli were delivered by two platinum wires applied to the outside of the axon. A typical intracellular action potential recorded by this method is shown in Figure 11. The resting potential is about −45 mV, and the over-

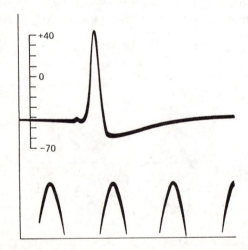

11

Intracellular recording of action potential from squid axon. Time base: 500 Hz. (From Hodgkin and Huxley, 1945.)

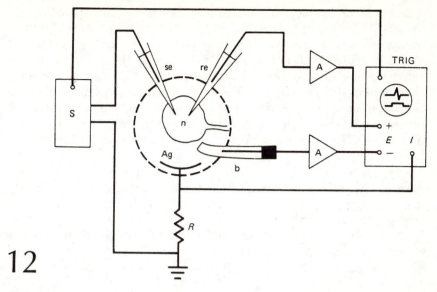

12

Experimental arrangement for intracellular recording from nerve or muscle fiber. n, nerve or muscle cell; E, transmembrane potential; TRIG, trigger signal. See text for more details.

SHOOT, or size of the positive phase measured from zero, is about +40 mV. The time base indicates that the action potential duration is about 0.7 msec. Also evident is the AFTER POTENTIAL, which follows the positive-going part of the spike. In the after potential the membrane potential is HYPERPOLARIZED, or made more negative than the resting potential, for about 2 msec. Action potentials in these single axons are ALL-OR-NONE; that is, once the stimulus reaches a certain level the action potential will occur, and no further increase in stimulus amplitude will change the form of the response.

In 1949, a more direct method of measuring membrane potentials in single muscle fibers was developed: Ling and Gerard pulled fine glass micropipettes, filled them with isotonic KCl, connected them to the recording amplifier, and stuck the electrodes right into living fibers. If the electrode tips were small enough (<0.5 μm), then membrane potentials could be measured for up to several hours. This method was soon adapted by Nastuk and Hodgkin (1950) for muscle fibers, and applied to many other preparations. A typical experimental arrangement for microelectrode work is shown in Figure 12. The preparation (in this case, a nerve cell body) is placed in a small recording chamber and covered with normal saline solution (a solution that approximates the natural extracellular fluid of the animal). Stimulating and recording electrodes (se and re) having resistances of 5 to 20 MΩ are inserted into the cytoplasm through the cell membrane. A bridge (b) filled with saline-agar gel serves as the external voltage reference electrode. In the gel lies the chlorided silver lead, which is thus protected from bumps and scrapes and changing ion concentrations around the preparation. Membrane potentials are measured differentially on the oscilloscope by subtracting the outputs of the preamplifiers (A). These preamplifiers must be direct-coupled and should have input impedances of at least 10^{10} Ω. The stimulator (S) applies current (I) between the stimulating electrode and ground. The return path for the current is through a chlorided silver wire in the bath (Ag) and series resistor (R). Injected current may thus be measured as the voltage drop across R.

To observe membrane responses with this arrangement, a trigger pulse is first produced, which starts the oscilloscope beam moving. Then a square stimulus pulse is applied to the cell. This produces a

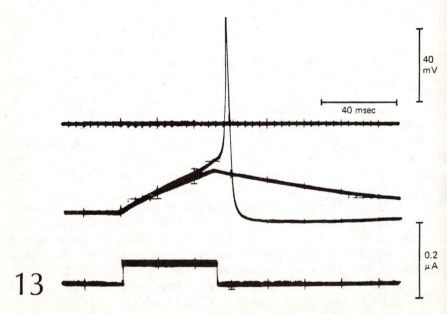

13

Action potential in an *Aplysia* neuron cell body. Upper trace, zero potential; middle trace, membrane potential; lower trace, current injected through membrane with intracellular microelectrode. Two sweeps superimposed, one in which the stimulus is subthreshold and one in which it is suprathreshold.

response such as that shown in Figure 13, taken from an *Aplysia* ganglion cell. The top trace shows zero potential, before the recording electrode was placed in the cell; each middle trace is membrane potential, and the bottom trace is injected current. Superimposed sweeps are shown, one in which the stimulus was too small to excite, and one in which it was just large enough. The threshold depolarization can be measured as that which is just large enough to excite. The resting potential was −48 mV and the overshoot was +56 mV. (How simple measurements such as these now seem, with our commercially available amplifiers and stimulators. Such data did not come as easily to the workers in the 1940s, but it was often first-rate in quality; c.f. Figure 11.)

OPTICAL RECORDING OF MEMBRANE POTENTIALS

In the early 1970s, several dyes were identified that, when applied to nerve membranes, showed an increased absorption of transmitted light during the action potential (Ross et al., 1974). This is illustrated in Figure 14 for the dye merocyanine applied to the squid axon. The bottom trace shows an action potential and the top trace shows the simultaneous decrease in transmitted light (increased absorption) at 570 nm. No signal could be recorded with the light source turned off, indicating that the optical recording was not due to electrical coupling between the action potential and the light-recording system. Also, no signal could be recorded in unstained axons, indicating that it was

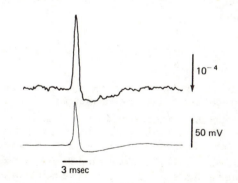

10^{-4}

50 mV

14

3 msec

Increase in light absorption during activity in squid axon stained with merocyanine dye. Top trace: Transmitted light (increasing downward) at 570 nm. Light calibration shows change in transmitted light divided by resting transmission. Bottom trace: Intracellularly recorded action potential. (From Ross et al., 1974.)

not due to some other optical effect such as light scattering. The signal-to-noise ratio with this method was high enough to permit accurate monitoring of spikes with single sweeps, in other words, averaging was unnecessary.

An early application of this technique was the simultaneous recording of activity from several neurons in a single invertebrate ganglion (Salzberg et al., 1977). This was accomplished by forming an enlarged image of the ganglion with a microscope objective and conducting the light from the images of single neurons to photodiodes with fiber-optic light guides. Nowadays, with smaller photodiodes, the light guides are omitted and arrays of up to 448 elements may be monitored at the same time (Nakashima et al., 1989). This technique allows us to observe the behavior of many elements of nervous structures during the performance of different behaviors. It thus gives a more accurate picture of the connections and interactions of the elements than was available with single-cell penetrations.

This has been a quick overview of extracellular and intracellular recording techniques. Both methods have been widely used. Extracellular recordings of single-neuron activity have been made almost everywhere in the brain of the cat. Intracellular recordings in mammals were first obtained in spinal motoneurons (Brock et al., 1952). This technique has been applied to a host of other classes of animals, which usually have larger, hardier cells than mammals. Recently, the PATCH PIPETTE METHOD has been used to study the activity of single ionic channels in nerve and muscle membranes. This technique, and the VOLTAGE CLAMP METHOD of controlling the membrane potential, will be discussed after we consider some other properties of resting and active membranes.

PROBLEMS

1. In Figure 5, calculate the conduction velocities of the fiber groups giving rise to the α and β peaks in the compound action potential.

2. In Figure 6, the conduction distance was 4 cm. Calculate the conduction velocities for the two peaks from the time between the stimulus artifact (small upward deflection at time 0) and the start of each elevation.

3. Using the conduction velocities in Problem 2 and the mean fiber diameters of each peak in the histogram in Figure 6, plot a two-point curve of velocity versus diameter. Estimate the slope of a straight line relating velocity and diameter.

4. The duration of the α deflection of the monophasic action potential in Figure 4 (about 1 msec) represents the time taken by the wave of activity in the nerve to pass by the recording electrode. If the wave is moving with the velocity found in Problem 1, what length of nerve is active during the action potential (or what is the wavelength of the action potential)?

5. In Figure 12, how large should the current-measuring resistor be to give a sensitivity on the current channel of the oscilloscope of a 10-mV deflection for a 100-nA injected current?

REFERENCES

Brock, L. G., Coombs, J. S. and Eccles, J. C. 1952. The recording of potentials from motoneurones with an intracellular electrode. *J. Physiol.* 117, 431–460.

Erlanger, J. and Gasser, H. S. 1937. *Electrical Signs of Nervous Activity.* Philadelphia, University of Pennsylvania.

Gasser, H. S. 1943. Pain-producing impulses in peripheral nerves. *Assoc. Res. Nerv. Ment. Dis., Proc.* 23, 44–62.

Hodgkin, A. L. and Huxley, A. F. 1945. Resting and action potentials in single nerve fibres. *J. Physiol.* 104, 176–195.

Hursh, J. B. 1939. Conduction velocity and diameter of nerve fibers. *Am. J. Physiol.* 127, 131–139.

Huxley, A. F. and Stämpfli, R. 1949. Evidence for saltatory conduction in peripheral myelinated nerve-fibres. *J. Physiol.* 108, 315–339.

Huxley, A. F. and Stämpfli, R. 1951. Direct determination of membrane resting potential and action potential in single myelinated nerve fibres. *J. Physiol.* 112, 476–495.

Julian, F. J., Moore, J. W. and Goldman, D. E. 1962a. Membrane potentials of the lobster giant axon obtained by use of the sucrose-gap technique. *J. Gen. Physiol.* 45, 1195–1216.

Julian, F. J., Moore, J. W. and Goldman, D. E. 1962b. Current-voltage relations in the lobster giant axon membrane under voltage clamp conditions. *J. Gen. Physiol.* 45, 1217–1238.

Ling, G. and Gerard, R. W. 1949. The normal membrane potential of frog sartorius fibers. *J. Cell. Comp. Physiol.* 34, 383–396.

Nakashima, M., Yamada, S., Shiono, S. and Maeda, M. 1989. A 448-channel optical monitoring of neural signals from *Aplysia* ganglion. *Soc. for Neurosci. Abst.* 15, 1046.

Nastuk, W. L. and Hodgkin, A. L. 1950. The electrical activity of single muscle fibers. *J. Cell. Comp. Physiol.* 35, 39–73.

Ross, W. N., Salzberg, B. M., Cohen, L. B. and Davila, H. B. 1974. A large change in dye absorption during the action potential. *Biophys. J.* 14, 983–986.

Salzberg, B. M., Grinvald, A., Cohen, L. B., Davila, H. V. and Ross, W. N. 1977. Optical recording of neuronal activity in an invertebrate central nervous system: simultaneous monitoring of several neurons. *J. Neurophysiol.* 40, 1281–1291.

Stämpfli, R. 1954. A new method for measuring membrane potentials with external electrodes. *Experientia* 10, 508–509.

Tasaki, I. and Takeuchi, T. 1941. Der am Ranvierschen Knoten entstehende Aktionsstrom und seine Bedeutung für die Erregungsleitung. *Pflügers Arch. Gesamte Physiol. Menschen Tiere* 244, 696–711.

Tasaki, I. and Takeuchi, T. 1942. Weitere Studien über den Aktionsstrom der markhaltiger Nervenfaser und über die elektrosaltatorische Übertragung des Nervenimpulses. *Pflügers Arch. Ges. Physiol. Menschen Tiere* 245, 764–782.

2

THE MEMBRANE ANALOGUE

ELECTRICAL PROPERTIES OF NEURON CELL BODIES

To describe the behavior of biological membranes, it is often convenient to employ electrical models, or analogues. These are approximations to the real membranes, but they have well-defined properties. Thus, we can say a resting nerve cell body behaves like a single-section RC circuit in response to an applied current. This is illustrated in Figure 1. The top shows the voltage response of an *Aplysia* nerve cell body to a subthreshold outward current pulse (same experimental arrangement as in Figure 12 of Chapter 1). The resting potential is about −45 mV; the outward current causes a depolarizing response since (+) charge is being passed from inside to outside the membrane by the intracellular stimulating electrode. Although the pulse of current is square, that is, the current is applied almost instantaneously, the curve of potential takes about 1 sec to reach its final value, near −38 mV. After the end of the pulse, a similar period of time is required for the potential to return to the resting level.

An electrical analogue that has the same type of response is seen in Figure 2. E_m is the total membrane potential at any time; E_r is the RESTING POTENTIAL; R_m is the MEMBRANE RESISTANCE; and C_m is a parallel MEMBRANE CAPACITANCE. If a current $I(t)$ is applied to this circuit, it will divide into two components: A current I_r will flow through the resistive branch, and I_c through the capacitative element, such that

$$I(t) = I_r + I_c \tag{1}$$

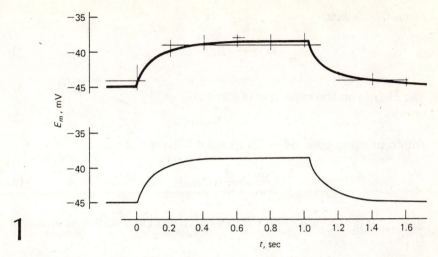

1

Comparison of nerve membrane response to square current pulse and that of a single-section *RC* filter. Top: Membrane potential of *Aplysia* neuron cell body. Bottom: Exponential response of a single-section filter designed to match the top response. Current step applied at time 0.

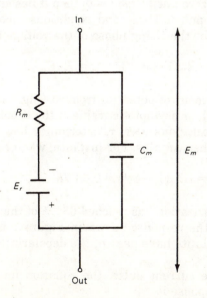

2

Single-section model of resting neuron cell body. The meaning of the abbreviations is found in the text.

From Ohm's law,

$$I_r = \frac{1}{R_m}(E_m - E_r)$$ (2)

The charge on the capacitor is given by

$$q = C_m E_m$$ (3)

Differentiating both sides of Equation 3 gives

$$\frac{dq}{dt} = \frac{d}{dt}(C_m E_m)$$ (4)

But dq/dt is the rate of flow of charge in the capacitative element, or I_c. So

$$I_c = C_m \frac{dE_m}{dt}$$ (5)

From Equations 1 and 2,

$$I(t) = \frac{1}{R_m}(E_m - E_r) + C_m \frac{dE_m}{dt}$$ (6)

The current stimulus is zero until time $t = 0$; then it has an amplitude i until the end of the pulse. These end conditions mean that the solution to Equation 6 for the rising phase of the voltage response is

$$E_m - E_r = iR_m(1 - e^{-t/\tau}) \qquad \tau = R_m C_m$$ (7)

$E_m - E_r$ is the displacement of potential from resting, in this case a depolarization. The final, or asymptotic, value of the depolarization is iR_m. The MEMBRANE TIME CONSTANT, τ, determines how rapidly E_m rises after the start of the stimulus. For instance, when $t = \tau$,

$$E_m - E_r = iR_m(1 - e^{-1}) = 0.632iR_m$$ (8)

By this time, the depolarization has reached 63.2% of the final value. The time constant for the response shown in Figure 1 is 0.124 sec. After several time constants have passed, the depolarization is quite close to iR_m.

After the end of the current pulse, the equation for the falling phase of the voltage response is

$$E_m - E_r = iR_m e^{-t/\tau}$$ (9)

Equations 7 and 9 are plotted in the bottom part of Figure 1 for comparison with the real membrane response.

Although the definitions R_m, C_m, E_m and τ apply, strictly speaking, only to the membrane analogue, they are freely transferable to the real cell for purposes of description. The usual method of measuring membrane resistance in a cell body is to apply a known current, i, for a long enough time that the potential change is essentially complete. Then R_m may be calculated as $(E_m - E_r)/i$. The time constant, τ, may be measured as the length of time required for $E_m - E_r$ to reach 63.2% of iR_m. The capacity, C_m, can then be calculated as τ/R_m.

CURRENT-VOLTAGE RELATION

This model is really only a first approximation to the cell membrane because R_m is not constant in most excitable cells but rather varies with membrane potential. This is a general electrical property called RECTIFICATION; it is illustrated in Figure 3. The abscissa shows the amplitude of current steps applied to an *Aplysia* neuron cell body, and the ordinate is the resulting change in potential. As the membrane is

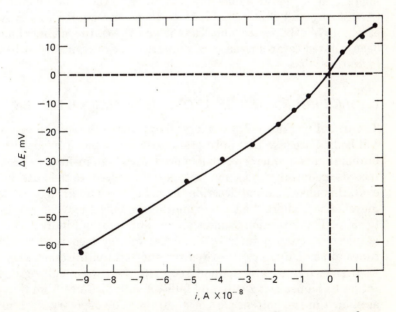

3

Resting current-voltage relationship of *Aplysia* neuron. Current steps of amplitude i applied through second intracellular electrode. ΔE measured from resting potential.

hyperpolarized (made more negative) or depolarized (made more positive) further than about 10 mV from resting, the curve starts to bend. If we remember that

$$R_m = \frac{E_m - E_r}{i} = \frac{\Delta E}{i} \tag{10}$$

then it is clear that R_m decreases from its value near the resting potential as the cell is strongly depolarized or hyperpolarized, because $\Delta E/i$ becomes smaller at potentials further than about 10 mV from resting. Near the resting potential, however, it is a good approximation to say that R_m is constant.

Almost all excitable cells show some sort of rectification over certain regions of membrane potential. For example, the squid axon shows a constant resistance in the hyperpolarizing direction and a relatively constant, but much lower, resistance in the depolarizing direction (Hodgkin et al., 1952). This behavior is known to result from an increase in potassium conductance with maintained depolarization. In frog skeletal muscle, however, the membrane resistance increases with depolarization (Adrian and Freygang, 1962). This property is called ANOMALOUS RECTIFICATION and is seen in certain cardiac muscle fibers and in squid axons injected with tetraethylammonium ions (Armstrong and Binstock, 1965). In these and other cases (Miyazaki et al., 1974; Hagiwara and Takahashi, 1974), the phenomenon has been related to an increase of potassium conductance with hyperpolarization.

CABLE PROPERTIES OF AXONS AND MUSCLE FIBERS

The model in Figure 2 gives a good approximation of the behavior of cell bodies because these are practically isopotential inside the membrane; that is, a microelectrode placed anywhere inside a neuron soma records essentially the same voltage with respect to the outside. However, this model cannot describe the behavior of an axon or vertebrate muscle fiber, where the transmembrane potential may vary from point to point. This situation is diagrammed at the top of Figure 4: A current is injected at the point $x = 0$ and the voltage measured at different times at some distance x away from the point of injection.

If a current step is applied at $x = 0$, then the resulting depolarization has a peak at $x = 0$, and falls off with distance from that point, as shown in the bottom part of Figure 4. (The depolarization is equal to $E_m - E_r$, the change from resting potential.) This illustrates the process of ELECTROTONIC CONDUCTION. In an axon or muscle fiber, po-

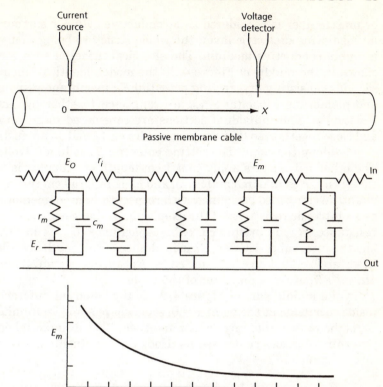

Current source

Voltage detector

Passive membrane cable

E_O r_i E_m In

r_m c_m

E_r Out

E_m

X

4

Electrotonic conduction in nerve or muscle fiber. Top: schematic of fiber with two intracellular microelectrodes; x = distance from stimulating electrode. Middle: electrical model of fiber; meaning of symbols is explained in text. Bottom: decline of final transmembrane potential, following application of a step current at $x = 0$, with distance x.

tential changes in one region are conducted to other parts of the cell by a purely passive mechanism. This process is DECREMENTAL, i.e., the signal falls off with distance, unlike the propagated action potential, which has a relatively constant amplitude. Electrotonic potentials are graded and vary with the stimulus amplitude, while the action potential is all-or-none.

CABLE THEORY

The simplest theory that can explain this behavior of axons and muscle fibers is called CABLE THEORY, as it was first worked out for transatlantic telegraph cables by Lord Kelvin (1855). In this view, the axon or muscle fiber is considered as a conductive cylinder surrounded by an insulating dielectric layer, the whole structure being immersed in a highly conductive medium. The electrical model of such a cable is shown in the middle of Figure 4. In the model, identical "membrane" sections consisting of a resting potential E_r, membrane resistance r_m, and membrane capacitance c_m are connected together by "internal" resistors r_i. The individual sections are considered to be very small and close together, so that the parameters r_m, r_i, and c_m are distributed evenly along the cable. The resting potential E_m is in millivolts (mV). The other parameters apply to a 1-cm length of cable; r_m is in ohm-cm ($\Omega \cdot$cm), r_i is in ohm/cm (Ω/cm), and c_m is in farad/cm (F/cm). These quantities may also be defined with respect to 1 cm^2 of membrane and as an intrinsic resistivity of the axoplasm. In that case, the membrane resistance, R_m, is in ohm-cm^2; the capacitance, C_m, is in farad/cm^2, and the internal resistivity, R_i, is in ohm-cm. The length-specific quantities are related to these by $r_m = R_m/\pi d$, $c_m = \pi d C_m$, and $r_i = 4R_i/\pi d^2$, where d = diameter of the cable.

In the middle part of Figure 4, E_0 is the potential difference from inside to outside at the point $x = 0$, somewhere along an infinite cable. E_m is the potential at any point x and time t. The differential equation governing E_m may be derived as (Hodgkin and Rushton, 1946)

$$-\lambda^2 \frac{\delta^2 E_m}{\delta x^2} + \tau_m \frac{\delta E_m}{\delta t} + E_m - E_r = 0 \qquad (11)$$

where $\lambda = \sqrt{r_m/r_i}$ is the membrane length constant
$\tau_m = r_m c_m$ is the membrane time constant

If a maintained current is applied to the core of the cable (as with a microelectrode), at the point $x = 0$ and starting at $t = 0$, then the voltage response of the cable at $x = 0$ is (Hodgkin and Rushton, 1946; Rall, 1960)

$$E_m - E_r = \Delta E_0 \, \mathrm{erf}\sqrt{t/\tau_m} \qquad (12)$$

where ΔE_0 = steady-state depolarization at $x = 0$
erf is the error function

When a sufficiently long time has passed after application of the current at $x = 0$, then a steady-state distribution of potential is reached along the cable. At this time $\delta E_m/\delta t = 0$, so Equation 11 becomes

$$-\lambda^2 \frac{d^2 E_m}{dx^2} + E_m - E_r = 0 \qquad (13)$$

The solution to this equation is

$$E_m - E_r = \Delta E_0 e^{-x/\lambda} \tag{14}$$

where ΔE_0 = steady-state depolarization at $x = 0$. In other words, the steady-state distribution of potential along a cable falls off exponentially with distance from the point of injection of current. This is shown on the bottom of Figure 4 for $t \to \infty$.

PROPAGATION OF THE ACTION POTENTIAL

It is this electrotonic coupling of nearby regions of an axon or muscle fiber that is responsible for propagation of the action potential. As shown in Figure 5, the transmembrane current in the active region is inward, as Na^+ ions flow from outside to inside. (This causes the internal potential to reverse, becoming positive in the active region, as mentioned in Figure 2 of Chapter 1.) But since charge is neither added to nor subtracted from the whole system, the inward current in the active zone must be balanced by an equal outward current in the neighboring inactive regions. We know from artificial injection of current with microelectrodes that outward current in an inactive region of membrane is depolarizing. Thus, the outward current in an inactive region that is produced by inward current in an active region depolarizes the inactive membrane to threshold and excites it. The sufficiency of this method of propagating the action potential was shown by Hodgkin in 1937; he demonstrated that action potentials that arrived at a crushed portion of nerve could depolarize the inactive nerve beyond the blocked area and could excite the inactive region if the block were small enough.

This type of analysis can also explain the variation of conduction velocity of action potentials with nerve fiber diameter: The internal

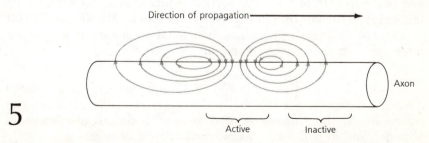

5

Propagation of action potential. Inactive region of axon or muscle fiber excited by local currents arising in the active zone. Further details in text.

resistance of the axons, r_i, through which the current must flow from active to inactive regions varies inversely with the square of the fiber diameter (see previous section). When r_i is lower, more current flows from the active to the inactive region, and the inactive region is more rapidly excited. This effect causes an increase in conduction velocity with increasing diameter (lower r_i). The membrane resistance, r_m, varies inversely with the first power of the diameter. However, it has an opposite effect from that of r_i: For a given amount of transmembrane current, a smaller r_m produces a lesser depolarization of the inactive region and excites it less rapidly. Since the effect of diameter is stronger on r_i, the conduction velocity varies approximately with the first power of fiber diameter. (An almost-linear relation between velocity and diameter was noted in Chapter 1.) The effects described by this analysis are equivalent to those of r_m and r_i on the length constant λ in Equation 11; the larger the length constant, the faster the conduction velocity.

EFFECTS OF MEMBRANE INFOLDING

The description of an axon or muscle fiber as a cylindrical cable is a useful first approximation but does not take into account the extensive infolding that often occurs in the walls of these cells. In muscle, the T-tubules, which are involved in excitation-contraction coupling, are continuous with the outside of the cell. This gives rise to charging curves with "creep," i.e., a slow potential response to a step of current that comes after the fast exponential component (Eisenberg and Gage, 1967, 1969). The giant axon of *Aplysia* (Figure 6) is riddled with folds of the surface membrane and is more ribbon-shaped than cylindrical for much of its length (Pinsker et al., 1976).

The effect of infolding is to increase the cell surface over that which would be expected for a non-infolded structure with the same cross-sectional area. This can be conveniently described with the area, A, and perimeter, P, of the cross section, which can be measured from micrographs such as that in Figure 6. As shown by Mirolli and Talbott (1972), the differential equation for axonal responses at long times after application of a current step at $x = 0$ is

$$-\left(\frac{A}{P} \cdot \frac{R_m}{R_i}\right) \frac{d^2 E_m}{dx^2} + E_m - E_r = 0 \qquad (15)$$

where R_m is the transverse resistance of 1 cm^2 of membrane in ohm-cm^2 and R_i is the axoplasmic resistivity in ohm-cm.

The solution of this is

$$E_m - E_r = \Delta E_0 e^{-x/(\sqrt{A/P}\sqrt{R_m/R_i})} \qquad (16)$$

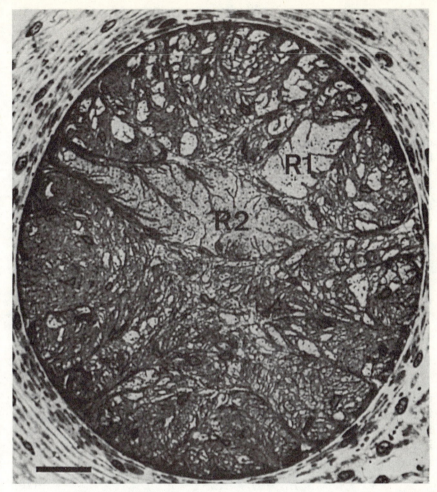

6   Light micrograph of a cross section of the right pleurovisceral connective
    in *Aplysia*. The largest axon is from the R2 cell and the next largest is
    from R1. Lead citrate stain. Calibration = 15 micrometers. (From Pin-
    sker et al., 1976.)

where ΔE_0 is the steady-state depolarization at $x = 0$.

Thus, by comparison with Equation 14, the length constant is

$$\lambda = \sqrt{\frac{A}{P}} \sqrt{\frac{R_m}{R_i}} \qquad (17)$$

For a cylindrical shape with diameter d, $A/P = d/4$; this applies to the value of λ in Equation 11 since, for a cylinder, $r_m/r_i = (R_m/R_i)(d/4)$. For other shapes, the value of λ depends on the geometrical quantity A/P. At a particular cross section A, increasing the amount of infolding increases the perimeter and shortens the length constant.

SOMA–AXON COUPLING IN REAL NEURONS

In real nerve cells, the electrical analogue that best describes the observed responses of the resting membrane is neither that of a cell body (soma) nor of an axon; it is both. In 1960 Rall described the theory for a lumped RC cell-body model connected to one end of an infinitely long axon cable. When a constant current is injected into the cell body with attached axon, the voltage response in the cell body is

$$E_m - E_r = \frac{\Delta E_0}{\alpha - 1} \left[\alpha \, \mathrm{erf}\sqrt{\frac{t}{\tau}} - 1 + e^{(\alpha^2 - 1)t/\tau} \, \mathrm{erfc} \, \alpha\sqrt{\frac{t}{\tau}} \right] \tag{18}$$

where ΔE_0 = steady-state potential change in cell body
$\quad\quad \alpha$ = ratio of axon end conductance to soma conductance
$\quad\quad \tau$ = time constant
$\quad\quad$ erf and erc are tabulated functions, erfc = 1 − erf.

This formidable expression may be simplified and applied to real nerve cells if we consider the significance of the parameter α: This number indicates the degree of dominance of the axon over the soma in giving rise to a certain voltage response. When $\alpha = 0$, the condition of very low axon end conductance or no coupling of the soma to the axon, then Equation 18 reduces to

$$E_m - E_r = \Delta E_0(1 - e^{-t/r}) \tag{19}$$

which is just the response of a single-section filter (Equation 7). When $\alpha \to \infty$, the condition of complete dominance by the axon, then Equation 18 becomes

$$E_m - E_r = \Delta E_0 \, \mathrm{erf}\sqrt{\frac{t}{\tau}} \tag{20}$$

as in Equation 12. Thus, by examining the shape of the charging curve of a neuron cell body, it is possible to estimate the degree of coupling of the cell body to axon or dendrite cable-like structures.

In Figure 7, the voltage response of an *Aplysia* neuron cell body (B) to an injected constant current is compared with Equation 19 (C) and Equation 20 (A). The value of α is apparently quite small and the

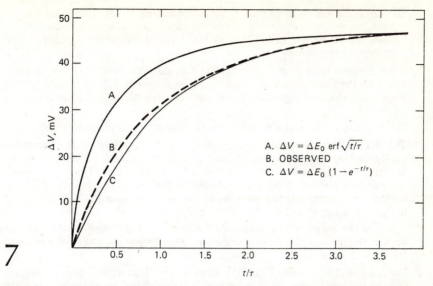

Analysis of degree of cable-like properties of *Aplysia* cell based on Rall theory. Curve A: Potential response of a semi-infinite cable to a current step. Curve B: Response of *Aplysia* cell. Curve C: Response of a single-section RC filter to the same stimulus. ($\Delta E_0 = 47.3$ mV.)

cell body itself seems to dominate the response (although the value of α depends strongly on the assumed time constant, τ; Junge, 1984). This situation should be contrasted with motoneurons in the cat spinal cord, which have a large number of attached dendrites with cable-like properties. Here, the value of α may be 25 or more, and the responses recorded in the cell body closely resemble those of a cable (Rall, 1959).

These electrical analogues of membranes have served a useful function in formalizing our ideas about nerve and muscle cells. However, it should be emphasized that they are based on constant parameters (i.e., are time- and voltage-invariant) and are thus an unrealistic view of living systems. In the following chapters, we shall see how the models can be expanded to account for such phenomena as nonlinearities in membrane I-V curves, and even for the action potential itself.

PROBLEMS

1. In the charging curve for a nerve cell membrane, given by Equation 7, how many time constants must elapse after the start of a square current stimulus before the depolarization ($E_m - E_r$) reaches 95% of the final asymptotic value (iR_m)?

2. The charging curve in Figure 1, top, is produced by an applied current of 9.2 nA. The time constant is 0.124 sec, and the asymptotic value of the depolarization is 6.7 mV. What is the total membrane resistance? The membrane capacitance?

3. If an *Aplysia* neuron cell body has the membrane resistance and capacitance in Problem 2 and is assumed to be a sphere 400 μm in diameter, what are the area-specific resistance (in $\Omega \cdot cm^2$) and capacitance (in $\mu F/cm^2$)?

4. What is the product of the area-specific resistance and capacitance?

5. The area-specific membrane capacitance in the *Aplysia* neuron may actually be the same as found in the squid axon, about 1 $\mu F/cm^2$. This can be calculated as in Problem 3, using a larger area than that of a sphere (probably a good assumption, because of the extensive infolding of the surface membrane). If the membrane capacitance is really 1 $\mu F/cm^2$, how many times larger is the area of the cell body than that of a sphere?

6. What is the corrected area-specific resistance for the *Aplysia* neuron cell body if the area is the above number of times larger than that of a sphere? (It is about 1000 $\Omega \cdot cm^2$ in the squid axon.)

7. Repeat Problem 1 using Equation 12 instead of Equation 7, that is, assuming the voltage response is that of the end of a cable. Choose the appropriate value of the error function from the following table:

Z	erf Z	Z	erf Z
0.90	0.797	1.20	0.910
0.95	0.821	1.25	0.923
1.00	0.843	1.30	0.934
1.05	0.862	1.35	0.944
1.10	0.880	1.39	0.950
1.15	0.896	1.45	0.960

8. In Mirolli and Talbott's (1972) study, the A/P ratio of a cross section of an infolded axon was measured as 9×10^{-5} cm. The diameter of a cylinder with the same cross-sectional area as this section of axon is 38 μm. What is the A/P ratio for this cylinder? What is the ratio of the axonal length constant to that expected for a cylinder with the same A, R_m, and R_i?

REFERENCES

Adrian, R. H. and Freygang, W. H. 1962. Potassium and chloride permeability of frog muscle membrane. *J. Physiol.* 163, 61–103.

Armstrong, C. M. and Binstock, L. 1965. Anomalous rectification in the squid axon injected with tetraethylammonium chloride. *J. Gen. Physiol.* 48, 859–872.

Eisenberg, R. S. and Gage, P. W. 1967. Frog skeletal muscle fibers: changes in electrical properties after disruption of transverse tubular system. *Science* 158, 1700–1701.

Eisenberg, R. S. and Gage, P. W. 1969. Ionic conductances of the surface and transverse tubular membranes of frog sartorius fibers. *J. Gen. Physiol.* 53, 279–297.

Hagiwara, S. and Takahashi, K. 1974. The anomalous rectification and cation selectivity of the membrane of a starfish egg cell. *J. Membr. Biol.* 18, 61–80.

Hodgkin, A. L. 1937. Evidence for electrical transmission in nerve, Part I. *J. Physiol.* 90, 183–210; Part II. *J. Physiol.* 90, 211–232.

Hodgkin, A. L., Huxley, A. F. and Katz, B. 1952. Measurement of current-voltage relations in the membrane of the giant axon of *Loligo*. *J. Physiol.* 116, 424–448.

Hodgkin, A. L. and Rushton, W. A. H. 1946. The electrical constants of a crustacean nerve fibre. *Proc. R. Soc. B* 133, 449–479.

Junge, D. 1984. Electrotonic coupling of soma and axon in the *Aplysia* R2 neuron. *J. Theor. Neurobiol.* 3, 97–112.

Kelvin, W. T. 1855. On the theory of the electric telegraph. *Proc. R. Soc.* 7, 382–399.

Mirolli, M. and Talbott, S. R. 1972. The geometrical factors determining the electrotonic properties of a molluscan neuron. *J. Physiol.* 227, 19–34.

Miyazaki, S., Takahashi, K., Tsuda, K. and Yoshii, M. 1974. Analysis of non-linearity observed in the current-voltage relation of the tunicate embryo. *J. Physiol.* 238, 55–77.

Pinsker, H., Feinstein, R., Sawada, M. and Coggeshall, R. 1976. Anatomical basis for an apparent paradox concerning conduction velocities of two identified axons in *Aplysia*. *J. Neurobiol.* 7, 241–253.

Rall, W. 1959. Branching dendritic trees and motoneuron membrane resistivity. *Exp. Neurol.* 1, 497–527.

Rall, W. 1960. Membrane potential transients and membrane time constant of motoneurons. *Exp. Neurol.* 2, 503–532.

3

IONIC PROPERTIES OF RESTING AND
ACTIVE MEMBRANES

ASYMMETRIC DISTRIBUTION OF IONS ACROSS THE MEMBRANE

The electrical analogues discussed in Chapter 2 provide a convenient description of the responses of real excitable membranes to applied stimuli. However, these models give no indication of the ions that are carrying the currents or of the molecular mechanisms of ion transport involved. One approach to this subject is the electrodiffusion theory of Nernst and Planck, which derives membrane potentials from asymmetric distributions of electrolytes across the cell membrane. This type of asymmetry is illustrated for squid axoplasm and blood in Table 1. It can be seen that the potassium ion concentration is much higher

Table 1. Approximate concentrations of ions in axoplasm and blood of squid, based on specific gravity of axoplasm and blood of 1.025 g/ml. (After Hodgkin, 1951.)

	Axoplasm, mmol/l	Blood, mmol/l
K^+	397	20
Na^+	50	437
Cl^-	40	556
Ca^{2+}	0.4	10
Mg^{2+}	10	54

inside the axon than outside and that the sodium and chloride concentrations are much higher outside. This situation could theoretically arise by at least two mechanisms.

There is in the axoplasm a sizable amount of negatively charged protein that cannot cross the membrane, and the resting membrane is mainly permeable to potassium and chloride. Thus, the K^+ and Cl^- could distribute in the directions shown in Table 1 according to a DONNAN EQUILIBRIUM. This mechanism is outlined in Figure 1. In this system, a membrane permeable to K^+ and Cl^- separates one compartment containing K^+ and Cl^- from another containing K^+, Cl^-, and an impermeant anion, A^-. For electroneutrality to exist in the outside solution,

$$[K]_o = [Cl]_o \tag{1}$$

and in the inside

$$[K]_i = [Cl]_i + [A] \tag{2}$$

Potassium has a tendency to move out of this membrane because it is more concentrated inside. But each K^+ ion that moves out must be accompanied by a Cl^- ion in order to maintain electroneutrality. This leads to an accumulation of Cl^- outside the membrane, which creates a concentration gradient opposite to that for K^+. These driving forces become equal at equilibrium, when the concentration ratios for the diffusible ions are equal; i.e.,

$$\frac{[K]_o}{[K]_i} = \frac{[Cl]_i}{[Cl]_o} \tag{3}$$

Taking $[Cl]_i$ from Equation 3 and substituting into Equation 2 gives

$$[K]_i = \frac{[K]_o}{[K]_i}[Cl]_o + [A] \tag{4}$$

1

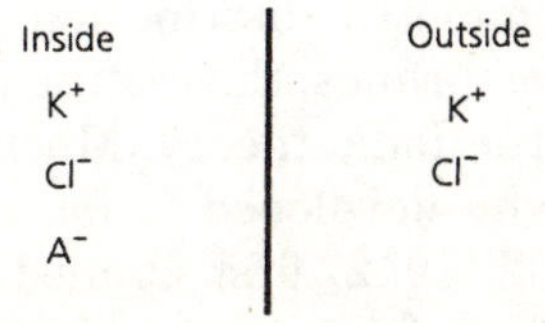

	Inside	Outside
	K^+	K^+
	Cl^-	Cl^-
	A^-	

Asymmetric ion distribution resulting from a Donnan equilibrium. A^-, impermeant anion.

Taking $[Cl]_o$ from Equation 1 and substituting into Equation 4 gives

$$[K]_i = \frac{[K]_o^2}{[K]_i} + [A] \tag{5}$$

or

$$[K]_i^2 = [K]_o^2 + [A][K]_i \tag{6}$$

So

$$[K]_i > [K]_o \text{ and } [Cl]_o > [Cl]_i \tag{7}$$

Equation 3 does not fit exactly with the data for K^+ and Cl^- in Table 1, but it does predict the proper directions of the change of K^+ and Cl^- concentrations from inside to outside. The K^+ and Cl^- concentrations inside and outside of frog muscle fibers follow a Donnan relationship quite closely. However, in this case an excess of impermeant sodium ions on the outside maintains the osmotic equilibrium (Boyle and Conway, 1941).

Another mechanism that operates in the excitable cell to accumulate potassium ions also acts to reduce the internal sodium ion concentration; this is the METABOLIC PUMP. As shown by Hodgkin and Keynes (1955), the squid axon membrane is continually extruding sodium ions from the inside to the outside by a process that requires adenosine triphosphate as an energy source. In addition, this sodium pump is coupled to the entry of potassium ions. If the external potassium is removed, the outward pumping of sodium is greatly reduced. Two potassium ions must enter for each three sodium ions that are pumped out (De Weer, 1984). Thus, the pump naturally functions to increase internal K^+ and reduce internal Na^+. As will be discussed in the next chapter, this type of pump operates in all known excitable cells, although the Na^+/K^+ coupling ratio may vary considerably from one system to another.

THE NERNST-PLANCK EQUATION FOR A SINGLE CATION

If one is given the asymmetric distribution of Na^+, K^+, and Cl^- ions across excitable cell membranes, the resting transmembrane potential may be derived from the ionic theory. Much of this theory is due to Nernst and Planck, who developed it for nonliving systems. Thus, though Bernstein (1902, 1912) first applied this theory to biological membranes, the equation for transmembrane potential in a single-electrolyte system is still called the Nernst equation. It may be derived easily for a system in which, for instance, the K^+ and Cl^- concentrations are different on two sides of a membrane. The membrane itself is assumed to play no role except to separate the two solutions; the calculation is really for the diffusion potential across the solution interface. First, the electrical potential is assumed to vary throughout the membrane (or the interface). Second, because the system is not in equilibrium, ION FLUXES will be present across the membrane. These fluxes each consist of two terms: one resulting from diffusional forces and the other from the effect of the membrane electric field on the charged ions. Thus, for the flux of potassium ion,

$$J_K = -D_K\left(\frac{d[K]}{dx} + [K]\frac{F}{RT}\frac{d\psi}{dx}\right) \tag{8}$$

where J_K = flux of K^+ in mol/sec/cm^2 of membrane
$\quad\ D_K$ = diffusion constant for K^+
$\quad\ \psi$ = potential at any point
$\quad\ F$ = Faraday constant
$\quad\ R$ = universal gas constant
$\quad\ T$ = temperature, K

This is referred to as the NERNST-PLANCK EQUATION for the flux of a single ion. Similarly, for the flux of chloride,

$$J_{Cl} = -D_{Cl}\left(\frac{d[Cl]}{dx} - [Cl]\frac{F}{RT}\frac{d\psi}{dx}\right) \tag{9}$$

With no net current imposed across the membrane, the currents due to K^+ and Cl^- should sum to zero, that is,

$$I = Z_K F J_K + Z_{Cl} F J_{Cl} = 0 \tag{10}$$

where I = total membrane current
$\quad\ Z$ = valence of ion
$\quad\ F$ = Faraday constant

So, substituting Equations 8 and 9 into Equation 10 gives

$$-D_K\frac{d[K]}{dx} + D_{Cl}\frac{d[Cl]}{dx} - \frac{F}{RT}\frac{d\psi}{dx}\left(D_K[K] + D_{Cl}[Cl]\right) = 0 \tag{11}$$

or

$$-\frac{F}{RT}\frac{d\psi}{dx} = \frac{D_K\dfrac{d[K]}{dx} - D_{Cl}\dfrac{d[Cl]}{dx}}{D_K[K] + D_{Cl}[Cl]} \tag{12}$$

A simplifying assumption is now made, that for electroneutrality, [K] = [Cl] at all points. Then

$$-\frac{F}{RT}\frac{d\psi}{dx} = \frac{(D_K - D_{Cl})\frac{d[K]}{dx}}{(D_K + D_{Cl})[K]} \tag{13}$$

This may be integrated directly as

$$\frac{F}{RT}(\psi_o - \psi_i) = \frac{D_K - D_{Cl}}{D_K + D_{Cl}} \ln \frac{[K]_o}{[K]_i} \tag{14}$$

If we now introduce the definition of MOBILITY as

$$u = \frac{D_K}{RT} \qquad v = \frac{D_{Cl}}{RT} \tag{15}$$

then Equation 14 becomes

$$E = \frac{u - v}{u + v}\frac{RT}{F} \ln \frac{[K]_o}{[K]_i} \tag{16}$$

where $E = \psi_o - \psi_i$ = transmembrane potential
$[K]_o$ = potassium concentration on outside
$[K]_i$ = potassium concentration on inside

If the membrane is now assumed to be permeable only to potassium, i.e., $v = 0$, then

$$E = \frac{RT}{F} \ln \frac{[K]_o}{[K]_i} \tag{17}$$

This expression for the potential across a membrane that is permeable only to one ionic species is often called the NERNST EQUATION. Because RT/F is about 25 mV at room temperature and $\ln([K]_o/[K]_i) \approx 2.3 \log([K]_o/[K]_i)$, Equation 17 predicts about a 58-mV change in potential for a tenfold increase in $[K]_o$. Figure 2 shows a fit of this equation to the variation of resting potential with external potassium concentration in frog muscle cells. The agreement is best at higher K concentrations; at lower values of $[K]_o$ the sodium permeability of the membrane makes the resting potential more positive than the theoretical line. However, the agreement with the Nernst-Planck theory is quite good.

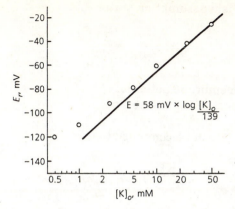

2

Variation of muscle fiber resting potential with external potassium ion concentration. Circles: membrane potential when external [K] was increased to the values shown in exchange for reduced [Na]. Straight line: Plot of Nernst equation (Equation 17). (After Adrian, 1956.)

THE GOLDMAN-HODGKIN-KATZ EQUATION

Bernstein's theory could account very well for the variation of resting potential with external potassium concentration, but it could not explain the inside-positive action potential observed by Hodgkin and Huxley (1939). The first step in modifying the ionic theory to embody this result was Goldman's work (1943), in which he related the membrane potential to the concentrations of several different electrolytes in the membrane itself. An assumption in his model was that the electric field, or rate of change of potential with distance, in the membrane, was a constant. Hence, his treatment is often referred to as CONSTANT-FIELD THEORY. This was used by Hodgkin and Katz (1949) to account for the membrane potential of squid axon. These authors performed many experiments in which they varied the external Na^+ and K^+ concentrations around the axons. They concluded, in agreement with Bernstein's theory, that the resting membrane was selectively permeable to potassium ions. However, in the active condition the squid axon membrane became selectively permeable mainly to sodium ions and not to all ions, as Bernstein had thought. This was reflected in the fact that the action potential overshoot varied only with external sodium concentration and was insensitive to potassium concentration.

The constant-field assumption states that

$$-\frac{d\psi}{dx} = \frac{E}{d} \qquad (18)$$

where E = transmembrane potential
$\quad\ d$ = thickness of the membrane

Equations 8 and 18 can be combined to give

$$\frac{d[K]}{dx} = -\frac{J_K}{D_K} + \frac{EF}{RTd}[K] \qquad (19)$$

This can be rearranged to give

$$\frac{d[K]}{-\dfrac{J_K}{D_K} + \dfrac{EF}{RTd}[K]} = dx \qquad (20)$$

Integration from 0 to d yields

$$\frac{RTd}{EF} \ln \frac{\dfrac{EF}{RTd}[K]_d - \dfrac{J_K}{D_K}}{\dfrac{EF}{RTd}[K]_0 - \dfrac{J_K}{D_K}} = d \qquad (21)$$

This can be solved for J_K as

$$J_K = \frac{D_K EF}{RTd} \frac{[K]_d - [K]_0 e^{EF/RT}}{1 - e^{EF/RT}} \qquad (22)$$

Now we can assume that the potassium concentrations in the membrane are proportional to those in the bulk solutions inside and outside:

$$[K]_d = \beta_K[K]_o; \qquad [K]_o = \beta_K[K]_i \qquad (23)$$

The current due to potassium is related to the flux by

$$I_K = FJ_K \qquad (24)$$

Defining the permeability P_K as

$$P_K = \frac{D_K \beta_K}{dF} \qquad (25)$$

we have

$$I_K = \frac{P_K E F^2}{RT} \frac{[K]_o - [K]_i e^{EF/RT}}{1 - e^{EF/RT}} \tag{26}$$

Similarly, for the currents due to sodium and chloride,

$$I_{Na} = \frac{P_{Na} E F^2}{RT} \frac{[Na]_o - [Na]_i e^{EF/RT}}{1 - e^{EF/RT}} \tag{27}$$

$$I_{Cl} = \frac{P_{Cl} E F^2}{RT} \frac{[Cl]_i - [Cl]_o e^{EF/RT}}{1 - e^{EF/RT}} \tag{28}$$

So the net current across the membrane is

$$I = \frac{EF^2 P_K}{RT} \frac{w - y e^{EF/RT}}{1 - e^{EF/RT}} \tag{29}$$

where $w = [K]_o + \dfrac{P_{Na}}{P_K} [Na]_o + \dfrac{P_{Cl}}{P_K} [Cl]_i$ (30)

$$y = [K]_i + \frac{P_{Na}}{P_K} [Na]_i + \frac{P_{Cl}}{P_K} [Cl]_o \tag{31}$$

When $I = 0$

$$w - y e^{EF/RT} = 0 \tag{32}$$

Then

$$E = \frac{RT}{F} \ln \frac{P_K[K]_o + P_{Na}[Na]_o + P_{Cl}[Cl]_i}{P_K[K]_i + P_{Na}[Na]_i + P_{Cl}[Cl]_o} \tag{33}$$

This is now conventionally referred to as the GOLDMAN-HODGKIN-KATZ EQUATION. Note that when $P_{Na}/P_K = 0$ and $P_{Cl}/P_K = 0$, the expression reduces to Equation 17, the Nernst equation.

By using Steinbach and Spiegelman's (1943) data for internal ion concentrations, Hodgkin and Katz (1949) found that the variation of the resting potential with potassium concentration could be accounted for if they assumed $P_K : P_{Na} : P_{Cl} = 1 : 0.04 : 0.45$. Furthermore, they could account for the internal-positive action potential quantitatively by assuming a 500-fold increase in sodium permeability in the active state to make $P_K : P_{Na} : P_{Cl} = 1 : 20 : 0.45$. This was an early analysis of the action potential mechanism, in which the membrane was thought to change from a mainly K^+- and Cl^--selective state to a mainly Na^+-selective state. This approach was soon replaced by the SODIUM HYPOTHESIS, in which the rising phase of the action potential was considered to result from an inflow of sodium ions through a specific Na^+-carrying system. The sodium hypothesis has now been verified by a number of independent methods, as will be discussed in Chapters 5, 6, 7, and 11.

CALCULATION OF CURRENT–VOLTAGE CURVE

The Nernst-Planck electrodiffusion theory can generate families of current-voltage, or I-V, curves that resemble those of the squid axon and other preparations under different ionic conditions. Thus, it has been widely applied in membrane biophysics. Equation 29 gives the predicted I-V relation under different internal and external ion concentrations. Although E is the independent variable, this equation also gives the I-V curve under conditions where a known current is injected and produces a potential change, since all the current is assumed to be carried by K^+, Na^+, or Cl^- ions. This is plotted in Figure 3, using the data of Eaton et al. (1975) for the *Aplysia* giant neuron. The resting potential at each external potassium concentration is the potential with zero injected current, which is the same as that predicted by Equation 33. Particularly at 10 mM external potassium, a strong curvature or rectification can be seen. This behavior is often referred to as CONSTANT-FIELD RECTIFICATION. This is a result of greater availability of internal K^+ for carrying outward currents than of external K^+ for carrying inward currents, and it practically disappears at higher external K^+ concentrations. This should be distinguished from rectification due to opening of membrane channels with changes in potential: The second type of rectification includes activation of inward current carrying channels by hyperpolarization, known as "anomalous rectification" (Chapter 2), and of outward channels by depolarization, known as "delayed rectification" (Chapter 5).

MEASUREMENT OF P_{Na}/P_K RATIO

It is possible to estimate the P_{Na}/P_K ratio in some excitable cells by using a simplified version of Equation 33. The term $P_{Na}[Na]_i$ is neglected as being much smaller than the terms to which it is added.

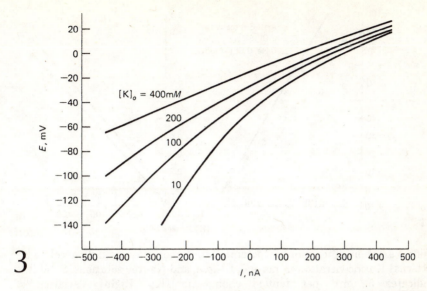

3

Current-voltage curves predicted by Nernst-Planck theory. External potassium concentrations in mM shown by each line. Data for *Aplysia* giant cell: $[K]_i = 280$mM, $[Na]_o = 485$, $[Na]_i = 61$, $[Cl]_o = 485$, $[Cl]_i = 51$, $P_{Na}/P_K = 0.12$, $P_{Cl}/P_K = 1.44$.

$P_{Cl}[Cl]_i$ is neglected for a reason that will be indicated, and the experiments are conducted in solutions free of chloride, making $[Cl]_o = 0$. Equation 33 then becomes

$$E = \frac{RT}{F} \ln \frac{[K]_o + P_{Na}/P_K[Na]_o}{[K]_i} \qquad (34)$$

and

$$e^{EF/RT} = \frac{[K]_o}{[K]_i} + \frac{P_{Na}/P_K[Na]_o}{[K]_i} \qquad (35)$$

In Figure 4, these equations are plotted against the external potassium concentration and compared with the real membrane potential of a molluscan ganglion cell (from Gorman and Marmor, 1970). On the left, the curve of potential versus $[K]_o$ in chloride-free solution (solid dots) is about the same as that in chloride-containing solution

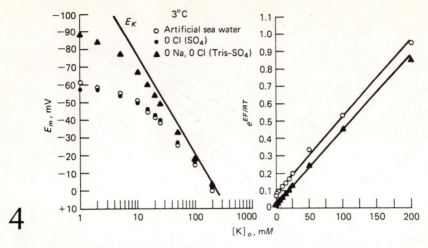

4

Left: Variation of membrane potential in a molluscan ganglion cell with external K concentration in normal, Cl-free, and Na-free solutions. Solid line indicates 58 mV per tenfold change in $[K]_o$. Right: Variation of $e^{EF/RT}$ with external K concentration. (From Gorman and Marmor, 1970.)

(open circles); thus, the resting membrane is relatively impermeable to chloride, justifying the dropping of $P_{Cl}[Cl]_i$ in Equation 33. Replacement of external sodium with Tris (tris-hydroxymethyl aminomethane, an impermeant cation, indicated here by triangles) causes the potential to follow the 58-mV line expected for a potassium-selective membrane much more closely. On the right of the figure, the values of $e^{EF/RT}$ agree well with Equation 35. When external sodium ion is replaced (triangles), the intercept changes and the slope is unaffected. The slope is equal to $1/[K]_i$, and the change in intercept is $P_{Na}[Na]_o/P_K[K]_i$. If one knows $1/[K]_i$ and $[Na]_o$, it is possible to calculate P_{Na}/P_K. Alternatively, the external potassium ion concentration may be held constant and $[Na]_o$ varied. In this case, the slope of the resulting line is $P_{Na}/(P_K[K]_i)$. The P_{Na}/P_K ratio is a useful description of a cell membrane at rest. It may also be applied to the active ionic channels, which, in addition to a large sodium ion permeability, do have some permeability to potassium.

ALKALI–CATION SELECTIVITY

A further description of the membrane channels is given by their alkali-cation selectivity, or their relative permeabilities to Li^+, Na^+,

K^+, Rb^+, and Cs^+. This measurement may be obtained by using a modified version of Equation 33: If a cation I^+ is the only external cation and chloride-free solutions are used, then the membrane potential becomes

$$E = \frac{RT}{F} \ln \frac{P_I/P_K[I]_o + P_{Cl}/P_K[Cl]_i}{[K]_i} \tag{36}$$

and

$$e^{EF/RT} = \frac{P_I/P_K[I]_o}{[K]_i} + \frac{P_{Cl}/P_K[Cl]_i}{[K]_i} \tag{37}$$

The internal chloride term is included because we have no a priori knowledge of how large it is. If the concentration of each cation is systematically changed, one at a time, then the graphs of $e^{EF/RT}$ versus $[I]_o$ should have slopes equal to $P_I/P_K[K]_i$. The value of $[K]_i$ may be obtained from the slope of the line when I^+ is K^+. Thus the relative permeabilities P_I/P_K may be found for all five cations.

Without any restricting assumptions, there are $5! = 120$ possible sequences of the five permeability ratios. However, with a very few exceptions, only 11 of these sequences are found in living or nonliving systems that bind cations. They are shown in Table 2. Sequence 1 is

Table 2. Observed sequences of alkali-cation selectivities. (From Eisenman, 1961.)

1.	Cs^+	>	Rb^+	>	K^+	>	Na^+	> Li^+
2.	Rb^+	>	Cs^+	>	K^+	>	Na^+	> Li^+
3.	Rb^+	>	K^+	>	Cs^+	>	Na^+	> Li^+
4.	K^+	>	Rb^+	>	Cs^+	>	Na^+	> Li^+
5.	K^+	>	Rb^+	>	Na^+	>	Cs^+	> Li^+
6.	K^+	>	Na^+	>	Rb^+	>	Cs^+	> Li^+
7.	Na^+	>	K^+	>	Rb^+	>	Cs^+	> Li^+
8.	Na^+	>	K^+	>	Rb^+	>	Li^+	> Cs^+
9.	Na^+	>	K^+	>	Li^+	>	Rb^+	> Cs^+
10.	Na^+	>	Li^+	>	K^+	>	Rb^+	> Cs^+
11.	Li^+	>	Na^+	>	K^+	>	Rb^+	> Cs^+

the lyotropic series, arranged in order of increasing hydrated size. Sequence 11 is arranged in order of increasing nonhydrated size. In the squid giant axon, sequence 4 describes the ionic dependency of the resting potential, and sequence 11 applies to the peak of the action potential. The other sequences are seen in various types of glass electrodes and in frog skin, frog and lobster muscle, *E. coli*, yeasts, red blood cells, *Chlorella*, crab nerve, and some enzymes (Eisenman, 1965).

EISENMAN THEORY

A simple, unifying theory that can explain this occurrence of only 11 out of 120 possible sequences was put forth by Eisenman (1961). The EISENMAN THEORY postulates that differences in anionic site strength in the membrane determine which of the 11 sequences is preferred in a given system. The argument goes as follows: In order for a cation in solution, I^+, to bind to a membrane site, S^-, it must first detach itself from the associated water molecule or molecules, W. The overall reaction is

$$I^+W + S^- \rightleftharpoons I^+S^- + W \qquad (38)$$

The standard free energy change for this reaction is

$$\Delta G_i^* = \Delta G_{\text{ion-site}} - \Delta G_{\text{ion-water}} \qquad (39)$$

At this point it is assumed that the most significant differences between $\Delta G_{\text{ion-site}}$ and $\Delta G_{\text{ion-water}}$ lie in the different electrostatic binding energies for the site and the water molecules. For a monovalent site, the binding energy is found from Coulomb's law as

$$\Delta U_{\text{ion-site}} = \frac{332q^+q^-}{r^+ + r^-} \qquad (40)$$

where $\Delta U_{\text{ion-site}}$ = binding energy, kcal/mol
q^+ = charge of the cation, electronic charges
q^- = charge of the anionic site, electronic charges
r^+ = crystal radius of the cation, Å
r^- = crystal radius of the anionic site, Å

The site strength may thus be varied by changing q^- or r^-. A smaller site permits a closer approach by a cation, which is thus more strongly bound. If, for instance, the radius of the anionic site is varied, then the binding energy $\Delta U_{\text{ion-site}}$ may be calculated for several different radii by using Equation 40. Values of the crystal radii and hydration energies for the alkali cations are listed in Table 3. We may thus calculate the overall change in binding energy for dehydration plus site binding as

$$\Delta U^* = \Delta U_{\text{ion-site}} - \Delta U_{\text{ion-water}} \tag{41}$$

This quantity actually gives the ion selectivity for each radius of the anionic site, because alkali cations with the most negative values of ΔU^* will be preferred. These are usually calculated with respect to a certain cation such as Cs^+; for instance,

$$\Delta U^R = \Delta U^*_{\text{ion}} - \Delta U^*_{\text{Cs}} \tag{42}$$

A sample calculation may elucidate this method: When $r^- = 3.5$ Å,

	Li^+	Na^+	K^+	Rb^+	Cs^+
$r^+ + r^-$, Å	4.28	4.48	4.83	4.99	5.15
$\Delta U_{\text{ion-site}}$, kcal/mol	−77.6	−74.1	−68.7	−66.5	−64.5
$\Delta U_{\text{ion-water}}$, kcal/mol	−24.2	−20.5	−15.8	−14.1	−12.7
ΔU^*, kcal/mol	−53.4	−53.6	−52.9	−52.4	−51.8
ΔU^R, kcal/mol	−1.6	−1.8	−1.1	−0.6	0

Table 3. Hydration energies and Goldschmidt crystal radii for the alkali cations. Hydration energies based on coulombic forces between single Rawlinson-type water molecules and each cation. (See Eisenman, 1961.)

	r^+, Å	$\Delta U_{\text{ion-water}}$, kcal/mol
Li^+	0.78	−24.2
Na^+	0.98	−20.5
K^+	1.33	−15.8
Rb^+	1.49	−14.1
Cs^+	1.65	−12.7

This is sequence 10, since the order of ion selectivities is $Na^+ > Li^+$ $> K^+ > Rb^+ > Cs^+$.

As the anionic site radius, r^-, is varied, different curves of ΔU^R versus r^- are produced for each cation, as shown in Figure 5. The size of ΔU^R represents the selectivity of the system (including ion-site binding and dehydration) for a particular ion as a function of anionic site radius. Because all the selectivities are referred to Cs^+, the ΔU^R for Cs^+ is invariant. However, as r^- is varied, the system selectivity changes through the 11 known sequences. At low anionic site radii (high site strength), Li^+ is preferred. A similar set of curves is obtained if the value of q^- is varied. Differences in anionic site strength could arise from inductive effects in membrane molecules (changing q^-) or from coordination effects, where several anionic sites are close enough to each other to interact with single cations.

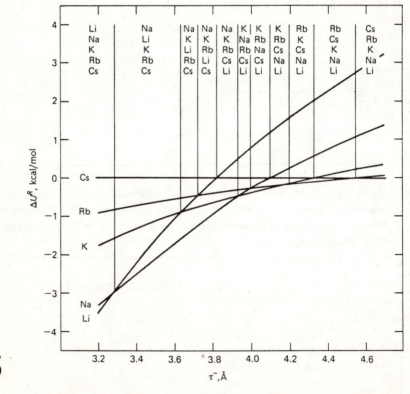

5

Theoretical variation of alkali-cation selectivity with membrane anionic site radius, r^-. ΔU^R, difference in energy site binding and dehydration relative to that for cesium. (Same method as Eisenman, 1961.)

Membrane selectivities for the halides, F^-, Cl^-, I^-, and Br^-, and for the divalent cations Sr^{2+}, Ba^{2+}, Ca^{2+}, and Mg^{2+} have also been calculated according to this theory and related to observed sequences (for review see Diamond and Wright, 1969). This powerful approach has explained many of the confusing properties of membranes, and it must be counted as a significant achievement of biophysical theory.

PARALLEL-CONDUCTANCE MODEL OF THE MEMBRANE

The Nernst-Planck electrodiffusion model of membrane ion fluxes has been widely applied to nerve and muscle cells because of its predictive strength. However, some of the assumptions used do not seem to apply to biological membranes (MacGillivray and Hare, 1969). For one thing, the assumption of electroneutrality (Equation 13) is not valid for a 100-Å membrane across which charge separation is known to exist (Agin, 1967). The theory predicts changes in potentials and I-V curves under different ionic conditions fairly closely, but is not applied to explain the transition from the resting to the active condition in an excitable membrane. Rather, the process of excitation of nerve and muscle is now thought to result from the sequential activation of independent sets of ion channels, each with its own particular selectivities (discussed in detail in later chapters).

Another approach to characterizing membrane ionic currents and the change from resting to active state is that of the PARALLEL-CONDUCTANCE MODEL, shown in Figure 6. This was described by Hodgkin

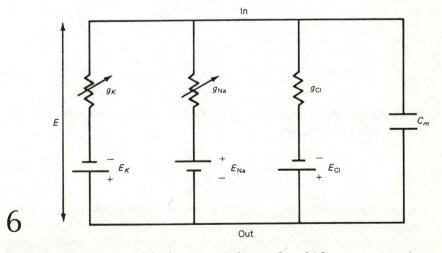

6

Parallel-conductance model of nerve membrane, for which one assumes independent conductance channels for K, Na, and Cl.

and Huxley (1952) and further elaborated by Hodgkin and Horowicz (1959). The membrane is thought to contain three parallel sets of channels, one for potassium ions, one for sodium ions, and one for chloride ions. Each set of channels is described by a battery, E, in series with a conductance, g (equal to the inverse of the resistance). The membrane capacitance, C_m, is across the whole ensemble. This model does not include longitudinal spread of current. Hence, it is only applicable to (1) small patches of membrane, (2) nodes of Ranvier, (3) axons in which a segment has been made isopotential with an internal electrode and external guards, or (4) nerve cell bodies where the inside is isopotential.

When $dE/dt = 0$—either at rest, at the peak of the action potential, or at the bottom of the after-potential—then the capacitative current ($C_m dE/dt$) disappears and all current flow is through the ionic channels, i.e.,

$$I = I_K + I_{Na} + I_{Cl} \tag{43}$$

or

$$I = g_K(E - E_K) + g_{Na}(E - E_{Na}) + g_{Cl}(E - E_{Cl}) \tag{44}$$

where E_K, E_{Na}, and E_{Cl} are the equilibrium potentials for each ion:

$$E_K = \frac{RT}{F} \ln \frac{[K]_o}{[K]_i} \tag{45}$$

$$E_{Na} = \frac{RT}{F} \ln \frac{[Na]_o}{[Na]_i} \tag{46}$$

$$E_{Cl} = \frac{RT}{F} \ln \frac{[Cl]_i}{[Cl]_o} \tag{47}$$

With no applied current, $I = 0$ and Equation 44 can be solved for the membrane potential as

$$E = \frac{E_K g_K + E_{Na} g_{Na} + E_{Cl} g_{Cl}}{g_K + g_{Na} + g_{Cl}} \tag{48}$$

In this formulation, g_{Na} is small compared to g_K in the resting membrane and increases during activity. The chloride conductance is usually considered to remain constant since replacement of external chloride with an impermeant anion does not affect action potentials or the associated currents. This model was used by Hodgkin and Huxley in reconstructing the squid action potential from theoretically obtained conductances (Chapters 5 and 6) and is also applied to describe post-synaptic responses to natural or chemical stimuli (Chapter 10).

EYRING RATE THEORY

An alternative theory of the membrane current-voltage relation is based on Eyring's theory of absolute reaction rates (Johnson et al., 1954; Eyring et al., 1964). This is a thermodynamic approach that describes the rate constants for chemical reactions in terms of energy barriers that must be overcome for the reactants to change into the products; hence, the formulations are often known as BARRIER MODELS.

A simple application of this theory to ionic interactions with membranes is that of the flux of a single cation, for which we shall use potassium. A three-barrier model of this process is shown in Figure 7. In part A, the solid curve is the standard chemical potential energy as a function of distance across the membrane. The left barrier (shown as peak on left) is the energy that must be overcome for a K^+ ion to leave the internal solution and associate with the membrane charge-carrying system. The middle barrier (large peak) is the energy of translocation across the membrane, and the right barrier is the energy of dissociation of the ion into the external solution.

For the left barrier, the forward rate constant for association, k_i, is given by

$$k_i = e^{-\Delta \mu_1 / RT} \tag{49}$$

where $\Delta \mu_1$ is the height of the barrier from the cytoplasmic side.

The backward rate constant, k_o, is

$$k_o = e^{-\Delta \mu_1^* / RT} \tag{50}$$

where $\Delta \mu_1^*$ is the height of the barrier from the adjoining well, and similarly for the other barriers.

In part B, the effect of an imposed transmembrane potential equal to $E = \Delta \Phi RT/F$ is shown. The broken line is the electrical potential energy profile and the solid curve is the total electrochemical potential energy, which is equal to the electrical plus the standard chemical energy. This figure illustrates the case in which the translocation barrier is much higher than the association barriers.

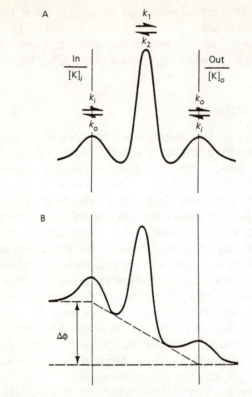

7

Three-barrier model of membrane potassium flux. Part A: Variation of standard chemical potential energy with distance. k_i = rate constant for association, k_o = rate constant for dissociation, k_1 and k_2 = rate constants for translocation. Part B: Total electrochemical potential energy under an applied depolarization of $E = \Delta\phi RT/F$.

The flux, J_1, of potassium ions across the left barrier, in mol/cm^2/sec, is

$$J_1 = [K]_i k_i - C_1 k_o \tag{51}$$

where $[K]_i$ is the potassium ion concentration in the internal solution
  C_1 is the concentration to the right of the barrier

If we assume that the rate constants for the right barrier are the same as for the left, then the flux across the right barrier is

$$J_3 = C_2 k_o - [K]_o k_i \tag{52}$$

where $[K]_o$ is the potassium concentration in the external solution
C_2 is the concentration to the left of the barrier

The flux across the middle barrier, J_2, is

$$J_2 = C_1 k_1 - C_2 k_2 \tag{53}$$

where k_1 and k_2 are the rate constants for the middle barrier.

Since an electrical potential energy equal to $\Delta\Phi/2$ is added to the standard chemical potential energy at the middle barrier (assuming a constant field in the membrane),

$$k_1 = e^{-(\Delta\mu_2/RT - \Delta\phi/2)} \tag{54}$$

$$k_2 = e^{-(\Delta\mu_2^*/RT + \Delta\phi/2)} \tag{55}$$

where $\Delta\mu_2$ and $\Delta\mu_2{}^*$ are the standard chemical potential energies of the center barrier measured from the adjoining wells.

So

$$J_2 = C_1 e^{-(\Delta\mu_2/RT - \Delta\phi/2)} - C_2 e^{-(\Delta\mu_2^*/RT + \Delta\phi/2)} \tag{56}$$

In this example, the standard chemical potential energy curve is symmetrical about the center of the membrane, so

$$\Delta\mu_2 = \Delta\mu_2^* \tag{57}$$

We can define a rate constant u_2 such that

$$u_2 = e^{-\Delta\mu_2/RT} \tag{58}$$

Then Equation 56 becomes

$$J_2 = C_1 u_2 e^{\Delta\phi/2} - C_2 u_2 e^{-\Delta\phi/2} \tag{59}$$

In the steady state $J_1 = J_2 = J_3 = J$, so

$$J = [K]_i k_i - C_1 k_o \tag{60}$$

$$J = C_1 u_2 e^{\Delta\phi/2} - C_2 u_2 e^{-\Delta\phi/2} \tag{61}$$

$$J = C_2 k_o - [K]_o k_i \tag{62}$$

Substituting for C_1 and C_2 in Equation 61,

$$J = \left(\frac{[K]_i k_i - J}{k_o}\right) u_2 e^{\Delta\phi/2} - \left(\frac{[K]_o k_i + J}{k_o}\right) u_2 e^{-\Delta\phi/2} \tag{63}$$

This can be solved for J as

$$J = \frac{[K]_i e^{\Delta\phi} - [K]_o}{\dfrac{k_o}{k_i u_2} e^{\Delta\phi/2} + \dfrac{1}{k_i} e^{\Delta\phi} + \dfrac{1}{k_i}} \tag{64}$$

If the middle peak in the chemical potential curve is much higher than the side peaks, then

$$u_2 \ll k_i \text{ and } k_o \tag{65}$$

So the left-hand term in the denominator of Equation 64 is much larger than the others, and J becomes

$$J = \frac{[K]_i e^{\Delta\phi} - [K]_o}{\dfrac{k_o}{k_i u_2} e^{\Delta\phi/2}} \tag{66}$$

We can now recognize that the transmembrane potential E is equal to $\Delta\Phi RT/F$, and the membrane current I is FJ:

$$I = \frac{F k_i u_2}{k_o} \frac{[K]_i e^{EF/RT} - [K]_o}{e^{EF/2RT}} \tag{67}$$

This gives the current-voltage relation for this system wherein the highest-energy step is translocation across the membrane. If the energies for association and dislocation with the membrane charge-carrying system are much higher than that for translocation, then Equation 64 becomes

$$J = \frac{[K]_i e^{\Delta\phi} - [K]_o}{\dfrac{1}{k_i} + \dfrac{1}{k_i} e^{\Delta\phi}} \tag{68}$$

and the current-voltage curve is

$$I = F k_i \frac{[K]_i e^{EF/RT} - [K]_o}{1 + e^{EF/RT}} \tag{69}$$

Equation 67 is plotted in Figure 8 for four different external potassium ion concentrations. At 10 mM K$^+$, the I-V curve is qualitatively similar to that predicted by the Nernst-Planck theory (shows outward rectification). At 200 mM K$^+$ (the same as the internal concentration), the curve is asymmetric about the zero-current point. At large values of $[K]_o$ this model shows inward rectification, i.e., increased conductance for large negative potentials. This behavior is not predicted by the Nernst-Planck theory but is seen in many excitable cells.

It must be remembered that Figure 8 shows only the currents due to a single cation and that an accurate description of a cell membrane must also have terms for sodium and chloride ions. These additional fluxes introduce assumptions about rate constants for association, dissociation, and translocation of Na^+ and Cl^- that are really unknown and cannot be easily measured.

The concept of cation selectivity also arises naturally from the Eyring approach: The right-hand energy barrier in Figure 7 can be equated with the difference in potential energies of the ion-water and ion-site interactions described under the Eisenman theory, above. This approach to selectivity theory is discussed in much more detail in a review by Krasne (1978). The barrier theory has also been applied to ion conductances in the squid axon (Woodbury, 1971), lipid bilayers (Hall et al., 1973; Läuger and Neumcke, 1973), and the node of Ranvier (Hille, 1975).

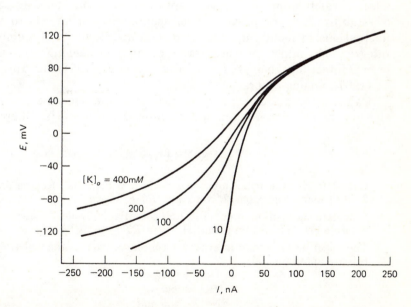

8

Potassium current-voltage curves predicted by Eyring rate theory. External potassium concentrations in mM shown by each line. Internal potassium concentration = 200 mM. $k_o = 100\ k_i u_2$.

Like the Nernst-Planck theory, the parallel-conductance model and the models of Eyring and others were formulated to explain membrane properties not predicted by earlier approaches. Each method has its own difficulties with the justification of underlying assumptions. But the vigorous application and exploration of the mathematical models has greatly enlarged our set of possibilities of what could be the case. This seems to be the usual process of development in a scientific field, where theory often precedes the available experimental techniques.

CALCIUM EFFECTS

The effects of calcium on nerve membranes were not covered by the Hodgkin-Katz paper in 1949, although some work had been done on the subject by that time (Arvanitaki, 1939; Brink et al., 1946; and Hodgkin, 1948). The usual result of lowering external calcium concentration in frog or squid nerve was to lower the critical, or threshold, depolarization for production of action potentials. In some cases, the neurons fired spontaneously in Ca-free solutions. Prolonged application of such solutions could lead to irreversible damage, a fall in membrane resistance, and subsequent inability to produce action potentials even with repeated washing in normal saline solution. The effect of calcium on nerve membranes was thus considered to be one of "stabilization," or prevention of spontaneous firing due to small fluctuations in membrane potential, and maintenance of membrane integrity. The importance of external calcium for keeping nerve membranes intact has been studied by Oomura et al. (1961) and Tasaki et al. (1967), among others.

Calcium can also substitute for sodium as the inward-current carrier in a variety of nerve and muscle cells; that story is for Chapter 8.

PROBLEMS

1. Calculate E_K, the potassium ion equilibrium potential, for the data in Table 1 using Equation 17. Note that $(RT/F) \ln x \approx 58 \log x$.
2. Calculate the sodium ion equilibrium potential in Table 1. Calculate the chloride ion equilibrium potential $E_{Cl} = (RT/F) \ln ([Cl]_i/[Cl]_o)$.
3. The major external and internal ion concentrations for the *Aplysia* giant cell are approximately

$$[K]_o = 10 \text{ m}M$$
$$[K]_i = 280 \text{ m}M$$
$$[Na]_o = 485 \text{ m}M$$
$$[Na]_i = 61 \text{ m}M$$
$$[Cl]_o = 485 \text{ m}M$$
$$[Cl]_i = 51 \text{ m}M$$

and the permeabilities for the resting membrane are in the ratios

$$P_K : P_{Na} : P_{Cl} = 1.0 : 0.12 : 1.44$$

What is the resting potential predicted by the Goldman-Hodgkin-Katz equation?

4. In Problem 3, what would be the effect on resting potential of a tenfold increase in external potassium ion concentration?

5. Using the data from Problem 3 and $P_K F^2/RT = 14.2$ (when E is in mV, I is in nA, and concentrations are in molarity), plot the potassium ion current in Equation 26 versus potential. Use potential as ordinate in 20-mV steps from -140 to $+60$ mV. Is there a noticeable constant-field rectification for the potassium current-voltage curve?

6. For the data in Figure 4, right side, the slopes of the lines of exp (EF/RT) versus [K] are both equal to 0.00426. From Equation 35, what is the predicted value of $[K]_i$?

7. In Problem 6, the external sodium ion concentration is 480 mM and the change in intercept on replacement of external sodium is 0.057. What is the P_{Na}/P_K ratio?

8. Calculate the selectivity sequence expected for cations when the radius of the anionic binding site is 4.4 Å.

9. In the parallel-conductance model of an *Aplysia* neuron, the relevant values for the resting membrane are

$$E_K = -83.9 \text{ mV}$$
$$E_{Na} = +52.2 \text{ mV}$$
$$E_{Cl} = -56.7 \text{ mV}$$
$$g_K = 0.177 \text{ } \mu\text{S}$$
$$g_{Na} = 0.116 \text{ } \mu\text{S}$$
$$g_{Cl} = 0.707 \text{ } \mu\text{S}$$

What is the predicted resting potential?

10. In Problem 9, what would be the effect on resting potential of a tenfold increase in external potassium ion concentration?

11. Find a simplified expression using a hyperbolic function for the current-voltage relation in Equation 67 when $[K]_i = [K]_o$.

12. Graph the current-voltage relationship for the three-barrier Eyring model with symmetrical potassium ion concentrations when the highest-energy steps are association and dissociation from the membrane charge carrier (Equation 69). Plot the potential as the ordinate in 20-mV steps from -140 to $+140$ mV, and assume that $k_i = 0.01$ and $[K]_i = [K]_o = 0.2 \text{ } M$.

REFERENCES

Adrian, R. H. 1956. The effect of internal and external potassium concentration on the membrane potential of frog muscle. *J. Physiol.* 133, 631–658.

Agin, D. 1967. Electroneutrality and electrodiffusion in the squid axon. *Proc. Natl. Acad. Sci. USA* 57, 1232–1238.

Arvanitaki, A. 1939. Recherches sur la réponse oscillatoire locale de l'axone géant isolé de «Sepia». *Arch. Int. Physiol.* 49, 209–256.

Bernstein, J. 1902. Untersuchungen zur Thermodynamik der bioelektrischen Ströme. *Pflügers Arch. Ges. Physiol. Menschen Tiere* 92, 521–562.

Bernstein, J. 1912. *Elektrobiologie.* Braunschweig, Vieweg u. Sohn.

Boyle, P. J. and Conway, E. J. 1941. Potassium accumulation in muscle and associated changes. *J. Physiol.* 100, 1–63.

Brink, F., Bronk, D. W. and Larrabee, M. G. 1946. Chemical excitation of nerve. *Ann. N. Y. Acad. Sci.* 47, 457–485.

De Weer, P. 1984. Electrogenic pumps: theoretical and practical considerations. *Electrogenic Transport: Fundamental Principles and Physiological Implications*, M. P. Blaustein and M. Lieberman (eds.), Society of General Physiologists Series, V. 38. New York, Raven, 1–15.

Diamond, J. M. and Wright, E. M. 1969. Biological membranes: the physical basis of ion and nonelectrolyte selectivity. *Annu. Rev. Physiol.* 31, 581–646.

Eaton, D. C., Russell, J. M. and Brown, A. M. 1975. Ionic permeabilities of an *Aplysia* giant neuron. *J. Membr. Biol.* 21, 353–374.

Eisenman, G. 1961. On the elementary atomic origin of equilibrium ionic specificity. *Symposium on Membrane Transport and Metabolism*, A. Kleinzeller and A. Kotyk (eds.). New York, Academic, 163–179.

Eisenman, G. 1965. Some elementary factors involved in specific ionic permeation. *Proc. 23rd Int. Congr. Physiol. Sci., Tokyo*, Amsterdam, Excerpta Med. Found., 489–506.

Eyring, H., Henderson, D., Stover, B. J. and Eyring, E. M. 1964. *Statistical Mechanics and Dynamics.* New York, Wiley.

Goldman, D. E. 1943. Potential, impedance and rectification in membranes. *J. Gen. Physiol.* 27, 37–60.

Gorman, A. L. F. and Marmor, M. F. 1970. Temperature dependence of the sodium-potassium permeability ratio of a molluscan neurone. *J. Physiol.* 210, 919–931.

Hall, J. E., Mead, C. A. and Szabo, G. 1973. A barrier model for current flow in lipid bilayer membranes. *J. Membr. Biol.* 11, 75–97.

Hille, B. 1975. Ionic selectivity, saturation, and block in sodium channels. *J. Gen. Physiol.* 66, 535–560.

Hodgkin, A. L. 1948. The local electric changes associated with repetitive action in a non-medullated axon. *J. Physiol.* 107, 165–181.

Hodgkin, A. L. 1951. The ionic basis of electrical activity in nerve and muscle. *Biol. Rev.* 26, 339–409.

Hodgkin, A. L. and Horowicz, P. 1959. Movements of Na and K in single muscle fibres. *J. Physiol.* 145, 405–432.

Hodgkin, A. L. and Huxley, A. F. 1939. Action potentials recorded from inside a nerve fibre. *Nature (Lond.)* 144, 710–711.

Hodgkin, A. L. and Huxley, A. F. 1952. Currents carried by sodium and potassium ions through the membrane of the giant axon of *Loligo*. *J. Physiol.*, 116, 449–472.

Hodgkin, A. L. and Katz, B. 1949. The effect of sodium ions on the electrical activity of the giant axon of the squid. *J. Physiol.* 108, 37–77.

Hodgkin, A. L. and Keynes, R. D. 1955. Active transport of cations in giant axons from *Sepia* and *Loligo*. *J. Physiol.* 128, 28–60.

Johnson, F. H., Eyring, H. and Polissar, M. J. 1954. *The Kinetic Basis of Molecular Biology.* New York, Wiley.

Krasne, S. 1978. Ion selectivity in membrane permeation. *Physiology of Membrane Disorders*. T. E. Andreoli, J. F. Hoffmann, and D. D. Fanestil (eds.). New York, Plenum, 217–241.

Läuger, P. and Neumcke, B. 1973. Theoretical analysis of ion conductance in lipid bilayer membranes. *Membranes: A Series of Advances (vol. 2)*, G. Eisenman (ed.). New York, Dekker, 1–59.

MacGillivray, A. D. and Hare, D. 1969. Applicability of Goldman's constant field assumption to biological systems. *J. Theor. Biol.* 25, 113–126.

Oomura, Y., Ozaki, S. and Maéno, T. 1961. Electrical activity of a giant nerve cell under abnormal conditions. *Nature (Lond.)* 191, 1265–1267.
Steinbach, H. B. and Spiegelman, S. 1943. The sodium and potassium balance in squid nerve axoplasm. *J. Cell. Comp. Physiol.* 22, 187–196.
Tasaki, I., Watanabe, A. and Lerman, L. 1967. Role of divalent cations in excitation of squid giant axons. *Am. J. Physiol.* 213, 1465–1474.
Woodbury, J. W. 1971. Eyring rate theory model of the current-voltage relationships of ion channels in excitable membranes. *Chemical Dynamics: Papers in Honor of Henry Eyring*, J. O. Hirschfelder (ed.). New York, Wiley, 601–617.

4

METABOLIC PUMPS AND MEMBRANE POTENTIALS

We have seen that, in nerve and muscle cells, the intracellular sodium concentration is regulated at a value less than one-tenth of that in plasma or interstitial fluid, and the potassium concentration is 20 to 50 times higher inside the cells than outside. This asymmetry is the basis for many cellular functions: Ions flow down their concentration gradients to produce action potentials, postsynaptic potentials, and sensory receptor potentials. The potential energy of the sodium gradient is also used to pump hydrogen ions (Moody, 1984) and calcium ions (Baker et al., 1967) out of cells. The ionic asymmetry is thus one of the major substrates for the functioning of eukaryotic cells: It is only because of differences in internal and external ion concentrations that nerves conduct, muscles contract, and glands secrete.

The principal means by which intracellular Na^+ is kept low and K^+ high is by the operation of the SODIUM-POTASSIUM PUMP. As shown by Hodgkin and Keynes (1953, 1954), Caldwell et al. (1960), and others, the active extrusion of sodium is partially coupled to the entry of potassium ions. The coupling ratio in the squid axon is three sodium ions pumped out for each two potassium ions pumped in, and the process requires metabolic energy derived from the hydrolysis of adenosine triphosphate (ATP).

ELECTROGENIC NATURE OF THE SODIUM–POTASSIUM PUMP

Because the coupling ratio for sodium-potassium exchange is greater than 1:1, a transmembrane current is produced by the operation of

58

the pump, which contributes a component of membrane potential under normal conditions. This is diagrammed in Figure 1. As shown on the left side, sodium ions enter the cell, and potassium ions leave, both during activity and at rest, by flowing down their concentration gradients. The pump mechanism serves to reverse these fluxes and maintain the ionic gradients. Since more sodium is extruded than the amount of potassium pumped in, a net outward flux is produced by the pump. This is symbolized by the current I_p in the electrical model on the right side of Figure 1. E_r and g_r are the resting potential and conductance of the membrane ionic channels. The pump is considered to be a zero-conductance current source since pump-blocking agents do not greatly affect the conductance of nerve membranes (Junge and Ortiz, 1978; Gadsby and Nakao, 1989). An inward current I_p must flow at all times across the ionic conductance g_r to balance the outward current produced by the pump. This inward current adds a pump-dependent component of membrane potential equal to I_p/g_r. Since the current across the membrane conductance is inward, the resulting change of potential is a hyperpolarization. When the pump is blocked, by cooling or application of a specific chemical blocking agent, a depolarization results.

As indicated in the model in Figure 1, the amount of membrane polarization that is added by the pump depends on the membrane conductance. Thus, the squid axon, which has a very large conductance (around 10^{-3} S/cm^2), has a small pump-dependent component of po-

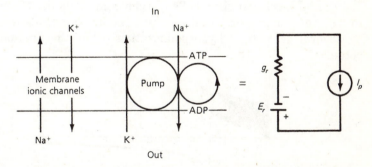

1

Mechanism of electrogenic sodium pump. Sodium and potassium, which enter and leave the cell through normal ionic channels (left) are actively pumped in opposite directions to their passive fluxes (center). Net active efflux of cations (I_p in diagram at right) causes equal and opposite current in ionic channels (E_r and g_r), producing a hyperpolarization that depends on g_r.

tential. Mollusc nerve cells, with smaller conductances (around 10^{-5} S/cm^2), show large pump-dependent potentials. In summary, the pump is electrogenic because it generates a net outward flow of cations through membrane areas other than the usual ionic channels; this is opposed by an inward flow of cations through the ionic channels, causing a hyperpolarization. While perhaps a bit oversimplified, this model is useful in understanding some of the phenomena produced in nerve and muscle cells by the actions of electrogenic pumps.

POSTTETANIC HYPERPOLARIZATION

One of the first such pump-related potential effects to be studied was posttetanic hyperpolarization (PTH). This consisted of a hyperpolarization of several millivolts, lasting for up to a minute after the end of a TETANUS, or burst of activity. It was first seen in sympathetic nerve trunks and peripheral nerves (Ritchie and Straub, 1957; Connelly, 1959; Straub, 1961; and Holmes, 1962). The membrane potentials of the fibers were measured across a sucrose gap that isolated an active region from an inactive region of membrane (see Chapter 1). A typical record of this behavior is shown in Figure 2, obtained with a cervical sympathetic trunk. The tetanus was produced by extracellular stimuli delivered to the trunk at 50 Hz for 5 sec. Immediately after the end of the tetanus, a hyperpolarization of about 3 mV was observed; it then decayed for several seconds.

During the next few years, further examples of PTH were found in the crayfish stretch receptor (Nakajima and Takahashi, 1966), rabbit vagus nerve (Rang and Ritchie, 1968; and Den Hertog and Ritchie, 1969), and leech ganglion cells (Baylor and Nicholls, 1969). All had in common the property that a burst of action potentials was followed by several seconds of hyperpolarization below the previous resting potential.

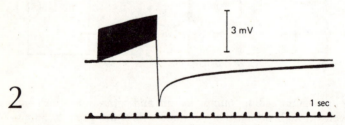

2

3 mV

1 sec

Posttetanic hyperpolarization in sympathetic nerve trunk. Black area caused by overlapping action potentials during tetanic (50-Hz) stimulation. (From Holmes, 1962.)

ELECTROGENIC PUMPS AND BLOCKING AGENTS

Two identified mechanisms that could give rise to the phenomenon of PTH are (1) stimulation of an electrogenic pump and (2) an increased conductance to ions with an equilibrium potential more negative than resting (probably K^+; the resting potential is usually somewhat more positive than E_K, because of the resting permeability to sodium and chloride).

All of the above examples of PTH have been shown to result from stimulation of electrogenic pump activity. Some of the evidence used in support of this conclusion included (1) that the PTH was reduced by lowering external K^+ concentration. This would be expected with a coupled pump, where external potassium is necessary for the Na^+/K^+ exchange to take place. It would not be expected for a K^+-conductance mechanism because lowering external potassium should make E_K more negative and increase the PTH. (2) The PTH was reduced or blocked by replacing external Na^+ with Li^+. Evidently, Li^+ could not be pumped out by the Na^+ pump and blocked the active extrusion of Na^+. (3) Agents (such as iodoacetate, azide, cyanide, and dinitrophenol) that interfered with the production of ATP, the energy source for the Na^+/K^+ pump, also blocked PTH. (4) PTH was reduced by ouabain or strophanthidin, which do not interfere with the production of ATP but block the active transport process in the membrane. (5) Cooling the preparation to 5 to 10°C strongly reduced the PTH, presumably by inhibiting the ATPase involved in the Na^+/K^+ exchange process. The effect of cooling was much larger than would be expected for a K-conductance mechanism. For instance, a Goldman-Hodgkin-Katz membrane potential (Equation 33, Chapter 3) would only become about 4% less negative upon cooling from 22 to 10°C, assuming the permeabilities did not vary with this temperature change.

Although all the above examples of PTH were shown to result from stimulation of electrogenic pumps, it should be mentioned that a K^+-conductance increase is responsible for the PTH seen in the node of Ranvier (Meves, 1961), phrenic motor nerve terminals (Gage and Hubbard, 1966), and *Aplysia* ganglion cells (Brodwick and Junge, 1972). However, this chapter is directed to the properties of electrogenic pumps, and not PTH per se.

STIMULATION OF ELECTROGENIC PUMPS

Hodgkin and Keynes (1956) demonstrated that injection of labeled Na^+ ions into squid axons stimulated active extrusion of sodium by the pump. The extrusion of Na^+ was proportional to the intracellular Na^+ concentration, suggesting that increasing the substrate acceler- ated the pump by mass action. In addition, Na^+ injection produced a small (1.6 mV) hyperpolarization, which was expected for an electro- genic (partially coupled) mechanism.

The first demonstration of an electrogenic pump in muscle (Kernan, 1962) also involved increasing the intracellular Na^+ concentration: Frog skeletal muscle was soaked in K^+-free solutions at low temper- atures; this blocked active Na^+ pumping and caused "loading" of the fibers with sodium. When the skeletal muscle was transferred to a recovery solution at room temperature with normal K^+ concentration, the membrane potentials became about 11 mV more negative than the calculated E_K. (This result stirred up some controversy because many investigators at the time considered the Na^+/K^+ pump in muscle to be completely coupled, and therefore neutral.) Then, in 1965, Mul- lins and Awad showed that Na^+-loaded muscles underwent a large hyperpolarization upon being warmed or transferred from a K^+-free to a high-K^+ medium, while muscles with a normal $[Na]_i$ did not. The next year it was shown (Adrian and Slayman, 1966) that Na^+-loaded muscle could attain membrane potentials 20 mV more negative than E_K, and that this hyperpolarization was abolished by ouabain. By 1966, the idea of an electrogenic pump in frog muscle was firmly established.

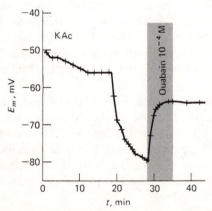

3

Effect of ouabain on Na-induced hyperpolarization in snail neurons. At time 0, potassium acetate injected. After about 20 minutes, sodium acetate injected. Ouabain added to external solution after injection of Na. (From Kerkut and Thomas, 1965.)

About this time, sodium injection was also shown to cause hyperpolarization in snail neurons by stimulation of an electrogenic pump (Kerkut and Thomas, 1965). The data of one such experiment are shown in Figure 3. At time zero, an electrode containing concentrated potassium acetate was inserted into the cell body; diffusion of KAc into the cell caused a slight increase in the resting potential, as would be expected for a K^+-permeable membrane. Twenty minutes later, an electrode filled with concentrated sodium acetate was inserted, and the membrane potential rapidly became 25 mV more negative. The effect of sodium injection was reversed by ouabain, indicating that the sodium injection had produced the hyperpolarization by means of a pump. Nakajima and Takahashi (1966) also observed a long-lasting hyperpolarization of the crayfish stretch receptor after electrophoretic injection of sodium citrate. Other studies have been performed with sodium injection in snail neurons and will be discussed in connection with measurement of pump currents.

For a number of years, there was some dispute about whether an electrogenic pump operated in the squid axon, perhaps because the changes in membrane potential produced by the pump were smaller than those observed in nerve cell bodies. However, De Weer and Geduldig (1973) carried out careful measurements of squid axon membrane potentials using a low-drift recording system. An average depolarization of 1.4 mV was produced by application of strophanthidin to the axons; the depolarization was larger in Na^+-loaded axons and was blocked by cyanide. This observation supported the idea that there were no truly neutral (completely coupled) pumps.

As mentioned in connection with sodium-loaded muscle fibers, warming can stimulate the action of electrogenic pumps. Some investigators have taken the approach of studying pumps in nerve cells principally by warming. For instance, Carpenter and Alving (1968) observed the behavior of the *Aplysia* giant (R2) cell shown in Figure 4. In part A, the cell was warmed from 5 to 21°C, and a hyperpolarization of 9 mV occurred. In part B, the same procedure was repeated in the presence of ouabain, producing a depolarization with superimposed action potentials instead of a hyperpolarization. The hyperpolarization in part A was thus apparently caused by an electrogenic pump, and it was suggested that the depolarization in part B resulted from an increase in membrane Na^+ conductance upon warming. Subsequently, Marchiafava (1970) studied the effects of warming on this cell in the presence of ouabain and concluded that warming increased both the resting g_{Na} and g_K, but increased g_{Na} more than g_K; Carpenter (1970) reached the same conclusion.

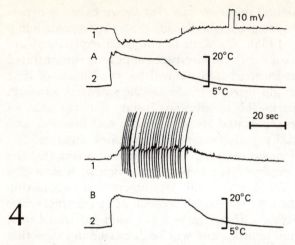

4

Effect of ouabain on the warming response of an *Aplysia* nerve cell. Top traces in A and B show membrane potential, bottom traces temperature near cell. Part A: Cell warmed from 5 to 21°C. Part B: Same warming with ouabain in external solution. (From Carpenter and Alving, 1968.)

Gorman and Marmor (1970) carried out a quantitative study of the effects of temperature and external potassium concentration on membrane potentials of *Anisodoris* neurons. The result of one of their experiments is shown in Figure 5. The open circles show the variation of exp (EF/RT) with external K^+ concentration at 5°C when the electrogenic pump is blocked. The straightness of this line is consistent with the constant-field expression for membrane potential (Equation 35, Chapter 3). The solid dots show the variation of exp (EF/RT) with $[K]_o$ at 18°C. Near $[K]_o = 0$ the pump is inhibited, and the potential is near that at 5°C. From about 5 to 50 mM $[K]_o$, the pump is activated, and the potential is more negative than that predicted by the constant-field equation. At higher values of $[K]_o$, the pump component of potential is small compared with that due to the passive ion conductances, and the curves at 5 and 18°C overlap. Thus, changes in ambient temperature do exert a strong influence on the metabolically derived component of potential. However, this method of controlling the pump action is not as specific as is the use of ouabain or strophanthidin because of the additional effect of temperature on the ionic conductances.

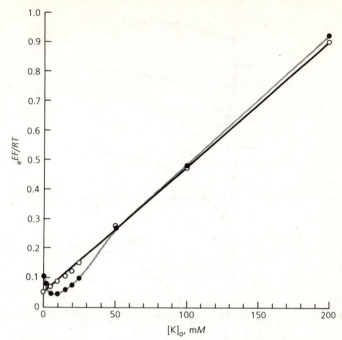

5

Effects of temperature and external K-concentration on electrogenic pump in mollusc neuron. Open circles: Variation of $e^{EF/RT}$ with $[K]_o$ at 5°C, when pump is blocked. Solid dots: Same measure at 18°C. Straight line shows constant-field variation of potential and K-concentration. (From Gorman and Marmor, 1970.)

VOLTAGE DEPENDENCE OF THE PUMP CURRENTS

The next step in analyzing electrogenic ion pumps came from the application of the voltage-clamp technique by Thomas (1969). This method is described in Chapter 5, and involves controlling the cell membrane potential with a feedback circuit. The current produced by the pump at a constant potential is then observed as shown in Figure 6. The start and end of injection of sodium acetate into a neuron cell body are indicated by downward- and upward-going marks near the start of each trace. Longer injections were used to increase the amount of injected sodium. Outward current, shown as a downward deflection, increased with increasing amounts of sodium injected. The remaining outward currents after the end of the injections declined with an

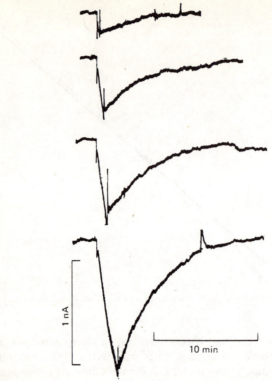

6

Sodium-pump currents measured with voltage clamp in snail neurons. (From Thomas, 1969.)

average time constant of 4.4 min. The pump currents were blocked by ouabain or potassium-free external solutions. This investigator also used intracellular sodium-sensitive microelectrodes to measure internal sodium concentration and found that the pump current was proportional to the excess of $[Na]_i$ over the normal level.

In 1972, Thomas extended these observations to the effect of membrane potential on the rate of sodium pumping. He used an intracellular Na^+-sensitive electrode to measure $[Na]_i$ under voltage-clamped conditions. The result was that hyperpolarization decreased the amount of Na^+ pumped out, as might be expected on energetic grounds, since the more negative potential provides a greater barrier for efflux of positive ions. About the same time, Kostyuk et al. (1972) looked at the effect of membrane potential on pump currents in response to Na^+ injection in snail neurons. They found that the outward current decreased with increasing hyperpolarization, although it was later suggested (Kononenko and Kostyuk, 1976) that this was due to an increased K^+ conductance during periods of high pump activity.

During the early 1980s, the weight of evidence continued to lean toward a voltage dependence of the pump (De Weer et al., 1988). Probably the first definitive study was done by Gadsby and Nakao (1989), using separated myocytes from guinea pig ventricles. Control of internal solutions was obtained with wide-tipped suction pipettes, and Cs^+ was substituted for potassium to block ionic currents through potassium channels. The external solution was sodium- and calcium-free. Pump currents were measured as the difference in voltage-clamp current produced by external application of strophanthidin. The voltage dependence of this current is shown in Figure 7. The outward current increases with a slightly sigmoid shape between −140 and 0 mV, starting to saturate at more positive potentials. This was the first *I-V* curve for the sodium pump obtained under conditions where all the ionic currents were blocked. Since the effect of the pump in an unclamped membrane is one of hyperpolarization, the voltage dependence of the pump may act as a kind of negative feedback.

PUMP REACTIONS

Ideas about the chemical mechanism of the transport process have been put forth since the 1950s (Skou, 1957; Rapoport, 1970; Glynn

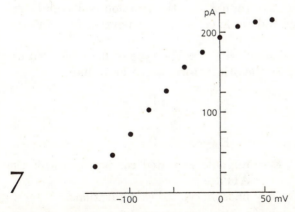

7

Current-voltage curve of Na/K pump in isolated ventricular myocytes. Ionic channel currents blocked; pump current measured as opposite of change in voltage-clamp current produced by strophanthidin. (From Gadsby and Nakao, 1989.)

and Karlish, 1975). However, little was known until recently about energetic properties such as the potential dependence of Na^+/K^+ exchange. One suggestive result was that of De Weer and Rakowski (1984), who were able to reverse the direction of pumping in the squid axon. Pump currents were measured as the change in voltage-clamp current when ouabain or another cardiotonic steroid was applied to the external solution; they were normally in the outward direction. When the internal fluid contained K^+ but no Na^+, and ADP instead of ATP, the pump current became inward, i.e., Na^+ was pumped in and K^+ out. The fluxes of Na^+ and K^+ running down their concentration gradients made the pump mechanism run backwards and synthesize ATP. This result led to the current concept of the relationship of ATP hydrolysis and movement of Na^+ and K^+ across membranes.

For a reversible pump mechanism, one can define an equilibrium potential, $E_{Na/K}$, at which the free energy of hydrolysis of ATP and the work required for the transfer of Na^+ and K^+ are equal and opposite (De Weer et al., 1988):

$$\Delta G_{ATP} + 3F(E_{Na} - E_{Na/K}) - 2F(E_K - E_{Na/K}) = 0 \qquad (1)$$

where F = Faraday constant
E_{Na} = sodium equilibrium potential
E_K = potassium equilibrium potential

Solving for $E_{Na/K}$,

$$E_{Na/K} = \Delta G_{ATP}/F + 3E_{Na} - 2E_K \qquad (2)$$

At potentials more negative than $E_{Na/K}$, the reaction is driven backwards, à la De Weer and Rakowski (1984), and generates a net inward current.

This reaction is consistent with a cyclic type of model, called an "Albers-Post" model, after the originators, which looks like

$$
\begin{array}{ccc}
E_1 & \longrightarrow & E_1\text{--}P \\
\uparrow & & \downarrow \\
E_2 & \longleftarrow & E_2\text{--}P
\end{array}
$$

where E_1, E_2 = unphosphorylated configurations of the ATPase
E_1–P, E_2–P = phosphorylated configurations

One ATP and three Na^+ bind to E_1 on the intracellular side of the membrane, forming E_1–P. This releases one ADP and changes to E_2–P, releasing Na^+ outside the cell and acquiring high affinity for K^+.

Two K^+ then bind to E_2–P, which changes to E_2 and releases K^+ intracellularly. E_2 then changes spontaneously back to E_1. This basic scheme has been modified to account for other known features of the Na^+/K^+ pump (Robinson, 1983; De Weer et al., 1988; Läuger, 1988).

MODEL OF THE UNSTIMULATED PUMP: THE MEMBRANE AT STEADY STATE

In order to explain the electrogenic effects of Na^+/K^+ exchange in nerve and muscle tissues, several models based on ion fluxes have been presented (Mullins and Noda, 1963; Moreton, 1969; Rapoport, 1970; Martirosov and Mikayelyan, 1970). The model of Mullins and Noda (1963) is the simplest that includes the effects of varying the Na^+/K^+ coupling ratio of the pump. It applies only to the steady-state condition of the membrane (potential or conductance not changing), and cannot account for potentials more negative than E_K, the potassium equilibrium potential.

The net passive flux of an ion into or out of the cell can be derived as

$$\overline{m} = P([C]_o - [C]_i e^{EF/RT})\, f(E) \tag{3}$$

where P = permeability of the ion
   $[C]_o$ = external concentration
   $[C]_i$ = internal concentration
   E = membrane potential
   R = universal gas constant
   T = temperature, K
   F = Faraday constant

The function $f(E)$ describes the potential dependence of the passive flux and is the same for any univalent ion. It is equal to $EF/[RT(1 - e^{EF/RT})]$ for the constant-field case but need not be stated in deriving this model.

It is assumed that only Na^+ and K^+ contribute to the resting membrane potential, chloride being distributed passively. The net passive influx of sodium, $\overline{m}_{Na}$, is balanced by an active efflux, $\overline{p}_{Na}$:

$$\overline{m}_{Na} + \overline{p}_{Na} = 0 \tag{4}$$

Similarly, for the passive efflux and active influx of potassium

$$\overline{m}_K + \overline{p}_K = 0 \tag{5}$$

If r is the number of sodium ions pumped out for each K^+ ion pumped in, then

$$r\bar{p}_K + \bar{p}_{Na} = 0 \tag{6}$$

Substituting from Equations 4 and 5 gives

$$r\bar{m}_K + \bar{m}_{Na} = 0 \tag{7}$$

From Equation 3,

$$rP_K ([K]_o - [K]_i e^{EF/RT}) f(E) + P_{Na} ([Na]_o - [Na]_i e^{EF/RT}) f(E) = 0 \tag{8}$$

This may be rewritten as

$$E = \frac{RT}{F} \ln \frac{rP_K [K]_o + P_{Na} [Na]_o}{rP_K [K]_i + P_{Na} [Na]_i} \tag{9}$$

If $r = 1$, that is, the outward flux of sodium is exactly equal to the inward flux of potassium, then Equation 9 becomes the Goldman-Hodgkin-Katz expression for the potential across a membrane permeable only to sodium and potassium. If r becomes infinite, the condition where no potassium ions are pumped out (zero net flux of K^+), then the potential becomes that of a potassium electrode. For intermediate cases, such as $r = 3$, the predicted potential is closer to the potassium equilibrium potential than for $r = 1$.

MODEL OF THE STIMULATED PUMP: THE MEMBRANE NOT AT STEADY STATE

In muscle cells that have been "sodium loaded" by soaking in low-K^+, high-Na^+ solutions, the sodium pump is abnormally active when normal saline solution is replaced around the cells. This may hyperpolarize the cell membrane to a potential more negative than E_K (Kernan, 1962; Adrian and Slayman, 1966) and may displace the membrane from steady state, causing both the potential and conductances to change with time. In order to describe this behavior, a constant efflux term can be added to the flux balance equation (Moreton, 1969):

$$\bar{m}_K + \bar{m}_{Na} + M_a = 0 \tag{10}$$

where $\bar{m}_K$ and $\bar{m}_{Na}$ have the same meaning as in Equations 2 and 3, and M_a = active efflux of cations.

Combining this with Equation 3 gives

$$-M_a = \frac{P_K EF}{RT} \frac{[K]_o - [K]_i e^{EF/RT}}{1 - e^{EF/RT}} + \frac{P_{Na} EF}{RT} \frac{[Na]_o - [Na]_i e^{EF/RT}}{1 - e^{EF/RT}} \tag{11}$$

This can be expressed as

$$E = \frac{RT}{F} \ln \frac{P_K[K]_o + P_{Na}[Na]_o + RTM_a/EF}{P_K[K]_i + P_{Na}[Na]_i + RTM_a/EF} \qquad (12)$$

Because some of the terms are found experimentally to be small compared to others, this equation may be simplified to

$$E = \frac{RT}{F} \ln \left[\frac{[K]_o}{[K]_i} + \frac{P_{Na}}{P_K} \frac{[Na]_o}{[K]_i} + \frac{RTM_a}{EFP_K[K]_i} \right] \qquad (13)$$

This is the same as the constant-field expression for a membrane permeable to sodium and potassium (Equation 34, Chapter 3), with the added pump term. Since E is negative in the resting cell, the pump term clearly acts as a hyperpolarization, i.e., reduces the argument of the logarithm. Since the membrane potential does not vary widely in the experiments described by Moreton (1969), the pump term may be considered approximately constant. M_a is assumed to approach zero when $[K]_o$ becomes zero, to account for Na^+/K^+ coupling. If M_a is sufficiently large, it is possible to reach membrane potentials more negative than E_K.

One can also construct Eyring-type models (Chapter 3) for the Na^+/K^+ pump mechanism, as the ions must be transported over electrochemical energy barriers to cross the membrane (Läuger, 1988). All of these formulations serve the same function as the Goldman-Hodgkin-Katz and Eyring theories do for resting nerve and muscle: they provide a theoretical basis for understanding the ionic properties of the excitable membranes involved.

DENSITY OF SODIUM PUMPING SITES

Ouabain or other glycosides labeled with tritium may be used to count the number of sodium-pumping sites per unit area in a particular biological membrane. This technique depends on the relatively tight binding of glycosides to the membrane ATPase, which is reflected in the difficulty of reversing the effects of these agents by washing a treated preparation with saline solution.

This method was first applied to whole and fractionated red blood cell ghosts (Hoffman and Ingram, 1969; Ellory and Keynes, 1969). The membranes were bathed in tritiated ouabain or digoxin, and the amount taken up was divided by an estimate of the membrane area. Assuming one molecule of glycoside binds to one Na^+-pumping site, these authors concluded that there is about one site per μm^2. Then Baker and Willis (1969) looked at ouabain uptake in a variety of cell cultures and found that the uptake by brain slices was more than 800 times as great as in red cell ghosts, implying a much larger number of pumping sites per unit area. Landowne and Ritchie (1970) confirmed the larger figure for nervous tissue and found an upper limit to the density of Na^+-pumping sites in rabbit vagus nerve of $750/\mu m^2$. This is necessarily an upper limit, since some of the labeled ouabain taken up by the axons may not be associated with the pumping sites. This density may be compared with the active Na^+-channel density of $75/\mu m^2$ found for this tissue by uptake of labeled TTX (Keynes et al., 1971). Baker and Willis (1972) estimated the density of sodium pumping sites in the squid axon as between $1,000$ and $10,000/\mu m^2$. In this preparation, the density of inward sodium channels has been found as $553/\mu m^2$ from binding of labeled TTX, and $312/\mu m^2$ from gating charge measurements (discussed in Chapter 7).

HYDROGEN ION PUMPING

As mentioned above, the sodium concentration gradient across excitable membranes has been shown to provide the energy for one type of extrusion of H^+ ions. It is known that these ions are normally removed from the cell by some transport process, since the cytoplasmic pH is more alkaline than that expected for an equilibrium distribution of H^+ at the resting potential (Moody, 1984). The distribution is given by

$$E = \frac{RT}{F} \ln \frac{[H^+]_o}{[H^+]_i} = \frac{RT}{F \log e} \log \frac{[H^+]_o}{[H^+]_i} \tag{14}$$

This is the same as

$$E = \frac{RT}{F \log e} (pH_i - pH_o) \tag{15}$$

Figure 8 shows the effect of removal of external sodium on the recovery of internal pH in a leech Retzius cell subjected to acid loading (Schlue and Deitmer, 1988). 20 mM NH_4Cl was added to the external solution for 1–2 min and then removed, which is known to cause a strong decrease in intracellular pH (Boron and De Weer, 1976). The right side shows the normal recovery of pH to a neutral value following this procedure, which takes about 10 minutes. As shown on the left side, when external sodium was replaced with the impermeant cation N-methyl-D-glucamine, the recovery was essentially blocked and the pH continued to fall. A similar result was obtained when amiloride,

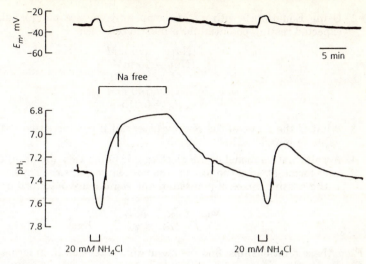

8

Sodium dependency of H^+ pump in leech Retzius cell. Top: membrane potential. Bottom: pH measured with intracellular electrode. Brief addition of NH_4Cl to external solution causes acidification of cytoplasm. Recovery from acidification (right side) is blocked in Na-free solution (left side). (From Schlue and Deitmer, 1988.)

which is known to interfere with sodium transport mechanisms, was applied in the external solution.

Thus, the transmembrane gradient of sodium is necessary for the maintenance of normal acidity in neurons, which also affects the synthesis and functioning of enzymes and other intracellular molecules. As mentioned in Chapter 8, the calcium efflux in excitable cells is also coupled to the sodium concentration gradient. So the fundamental, energy-requiring transport of sodium and potassium across membranes is the basis of a wide range of cellular functions, including excitability, which we shall now examine in detail.

PROBLEMS

1. In Equation 2, if the free energy of hydrolysis of ATP is -13.83 kcal/mol ($-57,900$ joules/mol) and the sodium and potassium equilibrium potentials are $+65$ and -95 mV, what is the reversal potential for the pump current, $E_{Na/K}$?

2. Using Equation 9 with $r = 1$ (completely coupled pump), calculate the expected resting potential for a muscle cell with

$$[\mathrm{Na}]_o = 115 \text{ m}M$$
$$[\mathrm{Na}]_i = 10 \text{ m}M$$
$$[\mathrm{K}]_o = 2.5 \text{ m}M$$
$$[\mathrm{K}]_i = 140 \text{ m}M$$
$$P_{\mathrm{Na}}/P_{\mathrm{K}} = 0.015$$

3. What is the value of the resting potential if r is increased to the typical value in muscle of 1.5?

4. An alternative model of the electrogenic pump uses the parallel-conductance formulation of the sodium and potassium currents. Thus, in Equation 7, the passive fluxes of potassium and sodium are described by

$$\overline{m}_{\mathrm{K}}F = I_{\mathrm{K}} = g_{\mathrm{K}}(E - E_{\mathrm{K}})$$
$$\overline{m}_{\mathrm{Na}}F = I_{\mathrm{Na}} = g_{\mathrm{Na}}(E - E_{\mathrm{Na}})$$

From these relationships, find the membrane potential, E, in terms of g_{K}, g_{Na}, E_{K}, E_{Na}, and r.

5. Using the result of Problem 4 when $r = 1$, find the resting potential for a muscle cell in which

$$E_{\mathrm{K}} = -101.4 \text{ mV}$$
$$E_{\mathrm{Na}} = 61.5 \text{ mV}$$
$$g_{\mathrm{K}} = 200 \text{ } \mu\mathrm{S/cm}^2$$
$$g_{\mathrm{Na}} = 17.6 \text{ } \mu\mathrm{S/cm}^2$$

6. Find the resting potential if r is increased to 1.5.

7. Using Equation 13 and the values below, calculate the resting potential of an *Aplysia* nerve cell when the sodium pump is blocked.

$$[\mathrm{K}]_o = 10 \text{ m}M$$
$$[\mathrm{K}]_i = 280 \text{ m}M$$
$$[\mathrm{Na}]_o = 485 \text{ m}M$$
$$P_{\mathrm{Na}}/P_{\mathrm{K}} = 0.12$$

8. Find the potential when the active efflux is sufficient to make

$$\frac{RTM_a}{EFP_{\mathrm{K}}[\mathrm{K}]_i} = -0.10$$

9. Landowne and Ritchie (1970) found an uptake of labeled ouabain to rabbit nerve of about 4.3 pmol/mg dry weight. If the membrane area is taken as 34 cm^2/mg dry weight, what is the density of ouabain-binding sites per square micrometer?

10. In some mouse muscle fibers, the internal pH has been measured as 7.2 (Aickin and Thomas, 1977). If the external pH is 7.4 and the membrane potential is -80 mV, what is the internal pH expected for an equilibrium distribution of H^+ ions? (At 37°C, the value of RT/F is about 26 mV.)

REFERENCES

Adrian, R. H. and Slayman, C. L. 1966. Membrane potential and conductance during transport of sodium, potassium, and rubidium in frog muscle. *J. Physiol.* 184, 970–1014.

Aickin, C. C. and Thomas, R. C. 1977. An investigation of the ionic mechanism of intracellular pH regulation in mouse soleus muscle fibres. *J. Physiol.* 273, 295–316.

Baker, P. F., Blaustein, M. P., Hodgkin, A. L. and Steinhardt, R. A. 1967. The effect of sodium concentration on calcium movements in giant axons of *Loligo forbesi*. *J. Physiol.* 192, 43–44P.

Baker, P. F. and Willis, J. S. 1969. On the number of sodium pumping sites in cell membranes. *Biochim. Biophys. Acta* 183, 646–649.

Baker, P. F. and Willis, J. S. 1972. Inhibition of the sodium pump in squid giant axons by cardiac glycosides: dependence on extracellular ions and metabolism. *J. Physiol.* 224, 463–475.

Baylor, D. A. and Nicholls, J. G. 1969. After-effects of nerve impulses on signalling in the central nervous system of the leech. *J. Physiol.* 203, 571–589.

Boron, W. F. and De Weer, P. 1976. Intracellular pH transients in squid axons caused by CO_2, NH_3, and metabolic inhibitors. *J. Gen. Physiol.* 67, 91–112.

Brodwick, M. S. and Junge, D. 1972. Post-stimulus hyperpolarization and slow potassium conductance increase in *Aplysia* giant neurone. *J. Physiol.* 223, 549–570.

Caldwell, P. C., Hodgkin, A. L., Keynes, R. D. and Shaw, T. I. 1960. The effects of injecting "energy-rich" phosphate compounds on the active transport of ions in the giant axons of *Loligo*. *J. Physiol.* 152, 561–590.

Carpenter, D. O. 1970. Membrane potential produced directly by the Na^+ pump in *Aplysia* neurons. *Comp. Biochem. Physiol.* 35, 371–385.

Carpenter, D. O. and Alving, B. O. 1968. A contribution of an electrogenic Na^+ pump to membrane potential in *Aplysia* neurons. *J. Gen. Physiol.* 52, 1–21.

Connelly, C. M. 1959. Recovery processes and metabolism of nerve. *Rev. Mod. Phys.* 31, 475–484.

De Weer, P. and Geduldig, D. 1973. Electrogenic sodium pump in squid giant axon. *Science* 179, 1326–1328.

De Weer, P. and Rakowski, R. F. 1984. Current generated by backward-running electrogenic Na pump in squid giant axons. *Nature (Lond.)* 309, 450–452.

De Weer, P., Gadsby, D. C. and Rakowski, R. F. 1988. Voltage dependence of the Na-K pump. *Annu. Rev. Physiol.* 50, 225–241.

Den Hertog, A. and Ritchie, J. M. 1969. A comparison of the effect of temperature, metabolic inhibitors and of ouabain on the electrogenic component of the sodium pump in mammalian nonmyelinated nerve fibres. *J. Physiol.* 204, 523–538.

Ellory, J. C. and Keynes, R. D. 1969. Binding of tritiated digoxin to human red cell ghosts. *Nature (Lond.)* 221, 776.

Gadsby, D. C. and Nakao, M. 1989. Steady-state current-voltage relationship of the Na–K pump in guinea pig ventricular myocytes. *J. Gen. Physiol.* 94, 511–537.

Gage, P. W. and Hubbard, J. I. 1966. The origin of the post-tetanic hyperpolarization of mammalian motor nerve terminals. *J. Physiol.* 184, 335–352.

Glynn, I. M. and Karlish, S. J. D. 1975. The sodium pump. *Annu. Rev. Physiol.* 37, 13–55.

Gorman, A. L. F. and Marmor, M. F. 1970. Contributions of the sodium pump and ionic gradients to the membrane potential of a molluscan neurone. *J. Physiol.* 210, 897–917.

Hodgkin, A. L. and Keynes, R. D. 1953. Metabolic inhibitors and sodium movements in giant axons. *J. Physiol.* 120, 46–47P.

Hodgkin, A. L. and Keynes, R. D. 1954. Movements of cations during recovery in nerve. *Symp. Soc. Exp. Biol.* 8, 423–437.

Hodgkin, A. L. and Keynes, R. D. 1956. Experiments on the injection of substances into squid giant axons by means of a microsyringe. *J. Physiol.* 131, 592–616.

Hoffman, J. F. and Ingram, C. J. 1969. Cation transport and the binding of T-ouabain to intact human red blood cells. *Proceedings of the First International Symposium on Metabolism and Membrane Permeability of Erythrocytes and Thrombocytes.* E. Deutsch, E. Gerlach, and K. Moser (eds.). Stuttgart, Thieme, 420–424.

Holmes, O. 1962. Effects of pH, changes in potassium concentration and metabolic inhibitors on the after-potentials of mammalian non-medullated nerve fibres. *Arch. Int. Physiol.* 70, 211–245.

Junge, D. and Ortiz, C. L. 1978. Measurement of electrogenic-pump current in *Aplysia* neurones with constant-current and constant-voltage techniques. *J. Exp. Biol.* 72, 141–151.

Kerkut, G. A. and Thomas, R. C. 1965. An electrogenic sodium pump in snail nerve cells. *Comp. Biochem. Physiol.* 14, 167–183.

Kernan, R. P. 1962. Membrane potential changes during sodium transport in frog sartorius muscle. *Nature (Lond.)* 193, 986–987.

Keynes, R. D., Ritchie, J. M. and Rojas, E. 1971. The binding of tetrodotoxin to nerve membranes. *J. Physiol.* 213, 235–254.

Kononenko, N. I. and Kostyuk, P. G. 1976. Further studies of the potential-dependence of the sodium-induced membrane current in snail neurones. *J. Physiol.* 256, 601–615.

Kostyuk, P. G., Krishtal, O. A. and Pidoplichko, V. I. 1972. Potential-dependent membrane current during the active transport of ions in snail neurones. *J. Physiol.* 226, 373–392.

Landowne, G. and Ritchie, J. M. 1970. The binding of tritiated ouabain to mammalian non-myelinated nerve fibres. *J. Physiol.* 207, 529–537.

Läuger, P. 1988. Electrogenic properties of the Na/K-pump. *The Ion Pumps: Structure, Function, and Regulation,* W. D. Stein (ed.). New York, Alan R. Liss, 217–244.

Marchiafava, P. L. 1970. The effect of temperature change on membrane potential and conductance in *Aplysia* giant nerve cell. *Comp. Biochem. Physiol.* 34, 847–852.

Martirosov, S. M. and Mikayelyan, L. G. 1970. Ion exchange in electrogenic active transport of ions. *Biofizika* 15, 104–111.

Meves, H. 1961. Die Nachpotentiale isolierte markhaltiger Nervenfasern des Frosches bei tetanischer Reizung. *Pflügers Arch. Gesamte Physiol. Menschen Tiere* 272, 336–359.

Moody, W. 1984. Effects of intracellular H^+ on the electrical properties of excitable cells. *Annu. Rev. Neurosci.* 7, 257–278.

Moreton, R. B. 1969. An investigation of the electrogenic sodium pump in snail neurones, using the constant-field theory. *J. Exp. Biol.* 51, 181–201.

Mullins, L. J. and Awad, M. Z. 1965. The control of membrane potential of muscle fibers by the sodium pump. *J. Gen. Physiol.* 48, 761–775.

Mullins, L. J. and Noda, K. 1963. The influence of sodium-free solutions on the membrane potential of frog muscle fibers. *J. Gen. Physiol.* 47, 117–132.

Nakajima, S. and Takahashi, K. 1966. Post-tetanic hyperpolarization and electrogenic sodium pump in stretch receptor neurons of crayfish. *J. Physiol.* 187, 105–127.

Rang, H. P. and Ritchie, J. M. 1968. On the electrogenic sodium pump in mammalian non-myelinated nerve fibres and its activation by various external cations. *J. Physiol.* 196, 183–221.

Rapoport, S. I. 1970. The sodium-potassium exchange pump: Relation of metabolism to electrical properties of the cell. I. Theory. *Biophys. J.* 10, 246–259.

Ritchie, J. M. and Straub, R. W. 1957. The hyperpolarization which follows activity in mammalian non-medullated fibres. *J. Physiol.* 136, 80–97.

Robinson, J. C. 1983. Kinetic analyses and the reaction mechanism of the Na,K-ATPase. *Curr. Top. Membr. Transp.* 19, 485–512.

Schlue, W.-R. and Deitmer, J. W. 1988. Ionic mechanisms of intracellular pH regulation in the nervous system. *Proton Passage Across Cell Membranes, Ciba Found. Symp. 139.* Chichester, Wiley, 47–69.

Skou, J. C. 1957. Influence of some cations on an adenosine triphosphatase from peripheral nerves. *Biochim. Biophys. Acta* 23, 394–401.

Straub, R. W. 1961. On the mechanism of post-tetanic hyperpolarization in myelinated nerve fibres from the frog. *J. Physiol.* 159, 19–20P.

Thomas, R. C. 1969. Membrane current and intracellular sodium changes in a snail neurone during extrusion of injected sodium. *J. Physiol.* 201, 495–514.

Thomas, R. C. 1972. Intracellular sodium activity and the sodium pump in snail neurones. *J. Physiol.* 220, 55–71.

5

VOLTAGE CLAMPING

MEASUREMENT OF MEMBRANE CURRENTS

By 1949, Hodgkin and Katz had a pretty good idea of how the nerve action potential worked. They were aware that the resting membrane was chiefly permeable to potassium and that an influx of sodium ions occurred during the action potential. The next step was to show quantitatively how ion movements gave rise to the observed action potentials. The major obstacle to this theoretical treatment was the difficulty of measuring the ionic currents directly. A large capacitive current, which was proportional to the rate of change of membrane potential, overlapped and masked the ionic part. To overcome this problem, Cole (1949) used a feedback circuit to hold the potential constant, eliminating the capacitive current. This device was known colloquially as the VOLTAGE CLAMP.

Hodgkin and Huxley were working with a similar system about the same time, and published an extensive analysis of their results in 1952. The method is outlined schematically in Figure 1. The membrane potential is measured between an internal silver wire and an external lead. A command signal, E_c, is added to the external potential at the input of the control amplifier. The output of the amplifier is fed back to the inside of the axon via an attenuator. When connected in the manner shown, the feedback acts to reduce the difference in amplifier inputs to zero, or make $E_i - (E_o + E_c) = 0$. But this also makes $E_i - E_o = E_c$, that is, transmembrane potential is made equal to E_c.

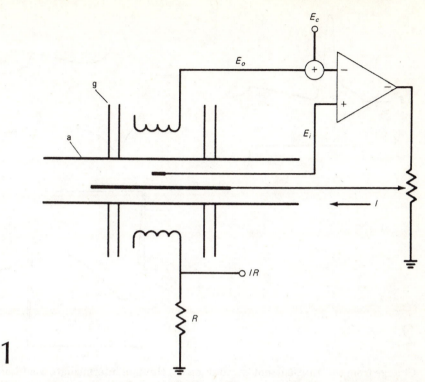

1

Voltage-clamp circuit for use with squid axon. a, axon; g, plastic guards. Uninsulated portion of internal voltage electrode indicated by short heavy line; uninsulated portion of current-injecting electrode indicated by long heavy line. E_i, internal potential; E_o, external potential; E_c, command potential. Feedback tends to make $E_i - E_o = E_c$. Injected current, I, measured as voltage drop across series resistor R.

The amount of current necessary to do this is measured across a series resistor from the bath to the circuit ground. Presumably, the injected current is equal and opposite to the current being generated by the nerve membrane. Usually a central portion of the nerve is insulated from the ends externally with plastic guards to limit the measured current to the area of membrane near the internal recording electrode. This method was developed by Marmont (1949) and eliminates the problems of longitudinal spread of current and spike propagation. With regular pulses applied at E_c, the membrane potential starts out looking like the top trace in Figure 2, part A: an action potential arising from a passive charging curve. The measured current has the

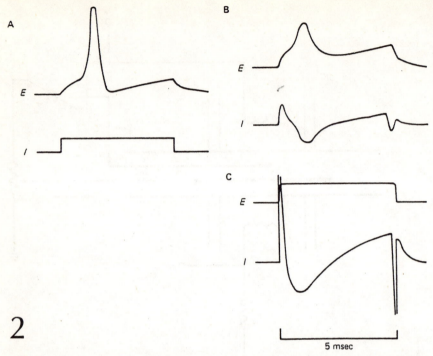

2

Change from constant-current stimulation (A) through intermediate condition (B), to voltage-clamp condition (C), as feedback in Figure 1 is increased. E, membrane potential. I, injected current.

same shape as E_c, a square pulse. As the feedback is turned up (part B), the potential record is somewhat flattened, and irregularities appear in the current record. With sufficient feedback, the potential record resembles E_c, and the current has the form shown in part C. The first peak is required to charge the membrane capacitance quickly and produce the square corner at the start of the potential record. Next, an inward current is observed (shown in the downward direction), followed by an outward current. At the end of the command pulse, a downward transient is seen as the membrane capacitance is suddenly discharged.

A series of currents measured in this manner in the squid axon by Hodgkin et al. (1952) is shown in Figure 3. These traces show injected currents following steps of potential from the resting level to the voltages shown on the right of each line. (Only the response to application of a command pulse is shown, not the response at the end of the command. The capacitive transients in Figure 2 have been removed, leaving gaps at time 0 in each trace.) At potentials more negative than −50 mV, little current is produced. Between −40 and about +40 mV, the direction of current flow is first inward through the membrane, then outward. Above +44 mV, the current is always outward.

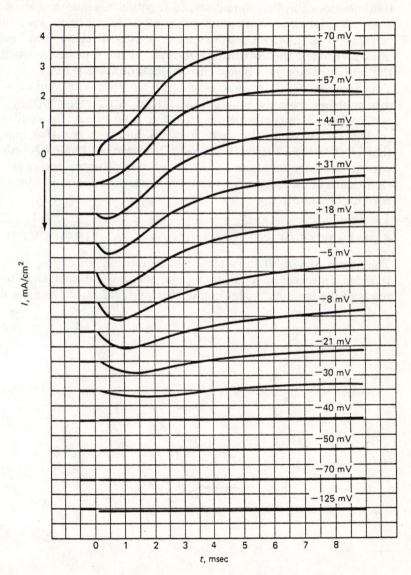

3

Currents measured with voltage clamp of squid axon. Inward currents indicated by downward deflections. Membrane held at about −60 mV (near resting potential), then stepped to potentials shown. (After Hodgkin et al., 1952.)

By measuring the currents at fixed times after the start of the command pulse, it is possible to construct *I-V* curves, such as the ones shown in Figure 4. The currents at 0.5 and 8 msec are plotted as functions of the level to which the membrane potential is stepped by the command pulse. The late currents clearly illustrate the rectification mentioned in Chapters 2 and 3; at potentials more negative than −40 mV, the conductance, or value of $\Delta I/\Delta E$, is very low; this is referred to as the LEAK CONDUCTANCE, because it arises from leakage of ions through the resting membrane. At more positive potentials, the late currents, and hence the conductance, are greatly increased. This phenomenon is known as DELAYED RECTIFICATION and should be distinguished from the constant-field rectification mentioned in Chapter 3, which is in the same direction but is not time-dependent.

The *I-V* curve for the early currents, however, is rather biphasic; that is, it falls and then rises again. Between −40 and +20 mV, the current actually decreases as the membrane potential increases. This characteristic is known as NEGATIVE RESISTANCE, and it indicates a region of instability.

SEPARATION OF SODIUM AND POTASSIUM CURRENTS

The above curves all show total membrane current during the nerve impulse. In order to separate out the sodium and potassium components of the current, Hodgkin and Huxley (1952a) did the experiment

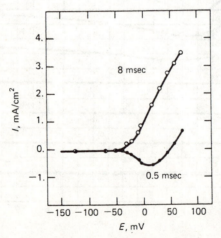

4

Current-voltage relation from voltage-clamp experiment in squid axon. (After Hodgkin et al., 1952.)

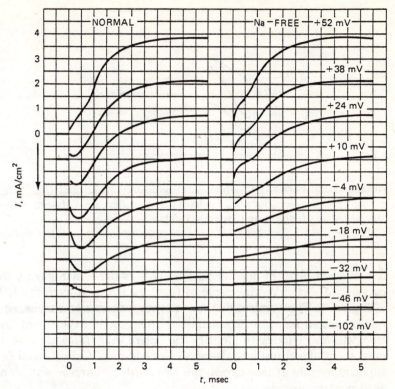

5

Currents measured in normal (left) and sodium-free solutions (right). Membrane potential held at −60 mV, then stepped to potentials shown on right. (After Hodgkin and Huxley, 1952a.)

whose data are shown in Figure 5. These traces are again currents (downward = inward) required to maintain the membrane potential at each level shown on the right, after stepping from the resting level (about −60 mV). The records on the left were obtained in normal saline, and those on the right in a solution in which all the sodium was replaced with choline. This cation maintained the normal osmotic pressure of the external solution, but it was presumably not able to cross the nerve membrane because of the large size of the molecule. The measured currents in the curves above +10 mV on the right side of the figure are carried by potassium and outward-moving sodium. At less-positive potentials there is little sodium outflow, and the outward-moving currents are equal to I_K. To obtain the variation of I_{Na} with time, the currents on the right are subtracted from those on the

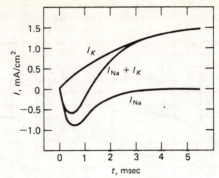

6

Voltage-clamp currents in squid axon measured in normal ($I_{Na} + I_K$) and sodium-free (I_K) solutions. I_{Na} calculated as difference between above two curves. (After Hodgkin and Huxley, 1952a.)

left at each level of depolarization. This is done in Figure 6 for the currents at -4 mV. The curve of $I_{Na} + I_K$ is taken from the left side of Figure 5. The vertical distance between these two curves, equal to I_{Na}, is plotted below for comparison. This type of experiment enabled Hodgkin and Huxley to identify the entire *early inward current* with movement of sodium ions. Because the curves of $I_{Na} + I_K$ and I_K were superimposable at late times, the *late outward current* was identified with potassium ions.

To describe these results, Hodgkin and Huxley used sodium and potassium conductances defined as follows:

$$g_{Na} = \frac{I_{Na}}{E - E_{Na}} \tag{1}$$

$$g_K = \frac{I_K}{E - E_K} \tag{2}$$

where

$$E_{Na} = \frac{RT}{F} \ln \frac{[Na]_o}{[Na]_i} \approx +60 \text{ mV} \tag{3}$$

$$E_K = \frac{RT}{F} \ln \frac{[K]_o}{[K]_i} \approx -70 \text{ mV} \tag{4}$$

The variation of g_{Na} and g_K with time following a step depolarization was similar to that of I_{Na} and I_K; that is, the sodium-carrying system first became conductive, and then the potassium system. The currents were considered to arise by flows of ions down their respective electrochemical gradients.

INSTANTANEOUS CURRENT-VOLTAGE RELATION

The above analysis suggests that the membrane follows Ohm's law and that a change in membrane current will be proportional to a change in potential. Of course, this test must be applied quickly after changing the potential because we know that conductances start to vary a few tenths of a millisecond after a depolarization. The type of measurement used by Hodgkin and Huxley (1952b) to confirm the assumption of linearity (i.e., conformity to Ohm's law) is called the INSTANTANEOUS CURRENT-VOLTAGE RELATION and is measured as shown in Figure 7. These data apply to the early inward (sodium) channels

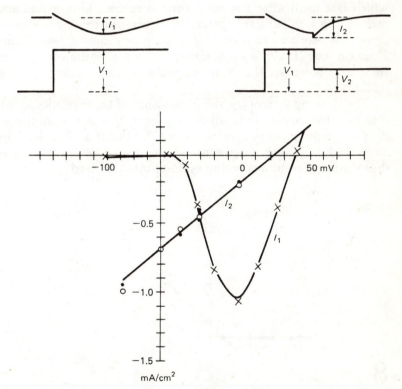

7

Instantaneous current-voltage relation obtained with voltage clamp for the early inward current. X's indicate normal peak inward currents for various depolarizations. Absolute membrane potential on abscissa; resting potential = −60 mV. Solid dots and circles indicate variation of I_2 with V_2 as shown in inset on right. Duration of first pulse = 1. 53 msec. (After Hodgkin and Huxley, 1952b.)

particularly. The first pulse of depolarization (V_1) activates the sodium channels and produces an inward current I_1. Now, with the sodium conductance turned on the potential is stepped to V_2. The purpose of this is to measure the change in current $I_2 - I_1$ as a function of the change in potential $V_2 - V_1$ while the sodium conductance is activated. The X's on the graph show I_1, the inward current at various values of V_1. The values of I_2 are plotted versus V_2, following a V_1 of 29 mV. However, the I_2 line reflects the change $I_2 - I_1$, because I_1 is the same for all values of I_2. It can be seen that I_2 varies linearly with V_2, and so the instantaneous *I-V* relation is in fact linear. Also of interest is the reversal of the "tail" of current, I_2, at a potential near E_{Na} (about +40 mV). This indicates that the "tail" currents are carried by sodium.

In Figure 8 the same experiment is repeated for long first pulses, which last until after the early inward current is over and activate mainly the late outward (potassium) current-carrying system. Once again, the result was a linear *I-V* relation for second pulses, confirming Hodgkin and Huxley's formulation of the potassium conductance. In this case, however, the "tail" currents reversed near E_K (at about −65 mV).

The striking symmetry and consistency of these results should not convince the reader that all nerves have linear instantaneous *I-V* curves; single nodes of Ranvier do not, for instance (Frankenhaeuser, 1960, 1963). In such cases a more complicated description of the sodium- and potassium-carrying systems must be used.

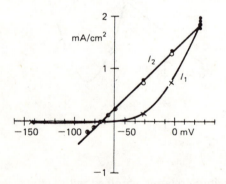

8

Instantaneous current-voltage relation for the late outward current. Same method as in Figure 7, but duration of first depolarization long enough for full development of outward current. X's show normal currents produced by first step of potential. Solid dots and circles show I_2 and V_2 as measured in Figure 7. (After Hodgkin and Huxley, 1952b.)

ACTIVATION AND INACTIVATION

As seen in Figure 6, the sodium current following a step depolarization has an initial peak and then drops off after a few milliseconds, unlike the potassium current, which builds up along a monotonic curve. Hodgkin and Huxley (1952c) considered that depolarization had two effects on the sodium current: ACTIVATION, or increased conductance, and INACTIVATION, which developed more slowly than the activation and "turned off" the current. To find the time course of inactivation, they carried out experiments such as that shown in Figure 9. This is a two-step voltage-clamp experiment in which the first conditioning depolarization is always 8 mV, and the second test pulse always brings the membrane potential to a level 44 mV more depolarized than its resting level. As the duration of the first pulse is increased, the inward

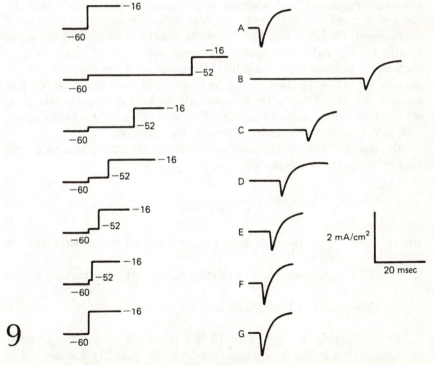

Time course of sodium inactivation. Left-hand column: Potentials under voltage-clamp conditions versus time. Right-hand column: Current versus time. (After Hodgkin and Huxley, 1952c.)

current in response to the second pulse begins to decrease. This inactivation develops with a half-time of a few milliseconds. If the first pulse is a hyperpolarization of 31 mV, the effect is a removal of the resting inactivation, as shown in Figure 10. In this case, the inward current in response to the second step of potential (44 mV more depolarized than when resting) is augmented above the one with no preceding pulse. Plots of development and removal of inactivation are shown in Figure 11. Both phenomena follow exponential curves, reaching maximal levels as the length of the first pulse is increased. The time constant of the inactivation in this figure is somewhat longer than that of removal of inactivation.

The voltage-dependence of inactivation of the sodium current is shown in Figure 12. This experiment had rather long (36 msec) conditioning pulses, so the effects developed maximally before the test pulses. With sufficiently large predepolarizations, as in A, the subsequent inward current in response to the test pulse was completely blocked; with no prepulse, as in E, a normal inward current was observed. Application of prehyperpolarization (F to I) augmented the inward current in response to the test pulse. To analyze this type of experiment, Hodgkin and Huxley made graphs such as that shown in Figure 13. The ratio of the inward current with each test pulse to that with no prepulse is plotted against the potential of the prepulse. Below about −90 mV, prepulses do not have much further effect on the test inward current. From −90 to −40 mV or so, the test current falls off sharply with increasingly positive prepulses. With those above −40 mV, the inward current is essentially blocked.

To describe this potential-dependent inactivation, Hodgkin and Huxley used an equation of the form

$$h = \frac{1}{1 + \exp\,[(V - V_h)/7]} \tag{5}$$

where h = a parameter that is proportional to the inward sodium current
V = depolarization of prepulse measured from resting potential
V_h = value of V at which $h = 1/2$

The smooth curve in Figure 13 is a plot of h versus the prepulse potential. This is the first paper in which the quantity h appeared in connection with sodium inactivation. It plays a major role in the subsequent theory of nerve excitation, and will be discussed in detail in Chapter 6.

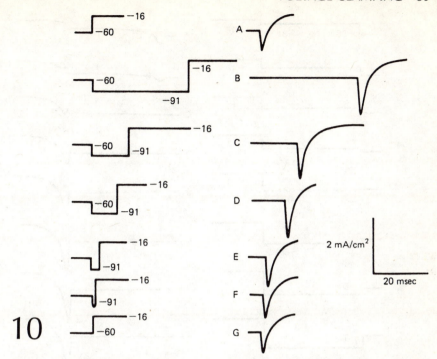

10

Time course of removal of resting sodium inactivation. Right and left columns show same measurements as in Figure 9. (After Hodgkin and Huxley, 1952c.)

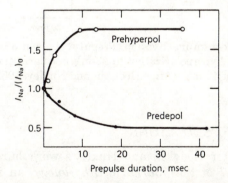

11

Time course of sodium inactivation. Curve marked PREDEPOL shows development of inactivation with conditioning depolarization of varying lengths. Curve marked PREHYPERPOL shows removal of resting inactivation with conditioning hyperpolarizations. Currents measured from data in Figures 9 and 10. (After Hodgkin and Huxley, 1952c.)

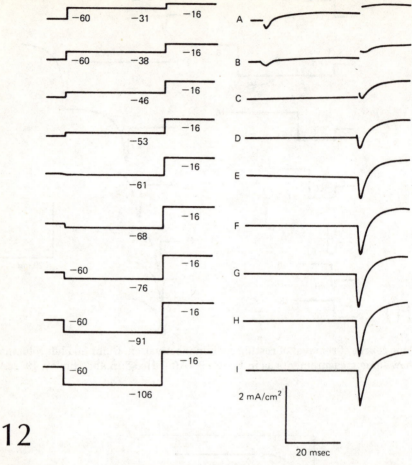

12

Voltage dependence of sodium inactivation. Prepulse of about 36 msec duration varied from 46-mV hyperpolarization to 29-mV depolarization, before a net test depolarization of 44 mV. (After Hodgkin and Huxley, 1952c.)

INTERNALLY PERFUSED AXONS

About nine years after Hodgkin and Huxley's work burst forth in volumes 116 and 117 of the *Journal of Physiology*, an interesting confirmation of their ionic theory was discovered: After squeezing the axoplasm out of squid giant axons with a roller, Baker et al. (1961) were able to reinflate the axons with solutions of their choosing. Action potentials such as that in Figure 14, top, could then be observed in the perfused axons for up to several hours. Among the observations made possible with this technique were that (1) in the presence of 10

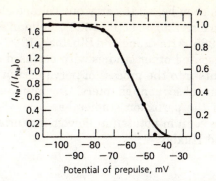

13

Voltage dependence of sodium inactivation. Normalized inward current in response to test pulse plotted against potential of conditioning pulse. Data from Figure 12. (After Hodgkin and Huxley, 1952c.)

mM external potassium the resting potential of the perfused axons varied about 58 mV per tenfold change in internal [K] except at the lowest internal concentrations, and (2) the action potential was blocked by increasing the internal sodium concentration to that of the external solution.

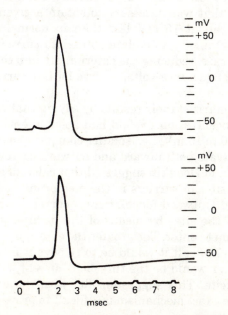

14

Action potentials in squid axon perfused with K_2SO_4 (top) and intact axon (bottom). (From Baker et al., 1961.)

Several laboratories then began to carry out voltage-clamp experiments using perfused axons (Moore et al., 1963; Adelman and Gilbert, 1964; Adelman et al., 1965; Armstrong and Binstock, 1965; and Tasaki and Singer, 1966). These and other studies with perfused axons have given many new insights into the process of nerve excitation, a topic that will be discussed in subsequent chapters. One might say that the most striking result of the perfusion studies has been the extent to which they confirm the sodium-potassium movements originally postulated by Hodgkin and Huxley.

EFFECTS OF CALCIUM ON MEMBRANE CURRENTS

The action of calcium on nerve membranes was first studied under voltage-clamp conditions by Frankenhaeuser and Hodgkin (1957), using the squid axon. They observed that reducing external calcium concentration caused a large increase in the inward current produced by a given depolarization. When they plotted peak sodium conductance, defined as in Equation 1, versus potential to which the membrane was stepped, they obtained the curves shown in Figure 15. Reducing the external calcium by a factor of 5 had the effect of shifting the conductance-voltage curve about 15 mV toward more negative potentials. That is, in low-calcium solutions the displacement of potential from resting that was necessary to obtain a given amount of inward current was about 15 mV less than in normal solution. A similar result was obtained for the late potassium current, as shown in Figure 16. In this case, reducing the external calcium concentration fivefold shifted the conductance-voltage curve for late current 10 to 15 mV more negative.

The authors summarized their results by saying that reducing the external calcium concentration fivefold had about the same effect as a depolarization of 10 to 15 mV; i.e., smaller changes in potential were then required to activate both inward and outward currents.

Frankenhaeuser and Hodgkin suggested that calcium might act by binding to negative sites or carriers in the membrane and exerting a stabilizing influence. Outward (depolarizing) currents would "wash" the calcium ions off the sites by means of the imposed electric field and thus allow sodium to enter. The greater the external concentration of calcium, the more difficult it would be to remove it from the membrane, and the greater would be the threshold current, or depolarization, required to excite. This suggestion fits with the experimental observations, but the exact mechanism is difficult to prove or disprove.

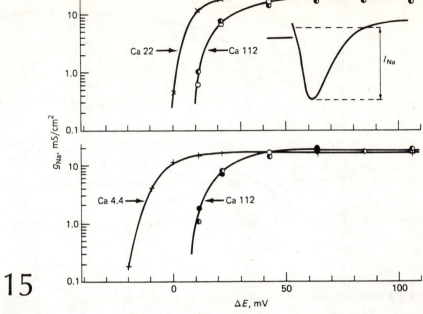

15

Effect of external calcium concentration on the variation of peak sodium conductance with membrane potential. (Calcium values next to curves show external concentrations.) Potential held at resting level, then displaced by the amount shown on the abscissa. (After Frankenhaeuser and Hodgkin, 1957.)

Blaustein and Goldman (1966) also measured shifts of the Na^+ conductance-voltage curve along the voltage axis with changes in the external calcium concentration. Hille (1968) published a curve of the variation of this shift with external calcium concentration in the node of Ranvier. Gilbert and Ehrenstein (1969), McLaughlin et al. (1971), D'Arrigo (1973), Brismar (1973), and others have suggested that calcium acts by forming a diffuse double layer outside the nerve membrane, which can affect the transmembrane electric field. This idea is summarized in Figure 17. The lower line shows the normal distribution of potential across a resting membrane. The potential does not change abruptly at the inner or outer surface but is smoothed out by microscopic changes in ion concentrations between the membrane and the bulk solutions. Within the membrane, the rate of change of potential with distance, or FIELD STRENGTH, is assumed constant. The CRITICAL GRADIENT, or field strength required to produce an action poten-

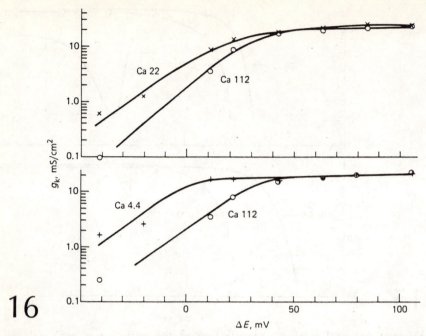

16

Effect of external calcium concentration on the variation of steady-state potassium conductance with membrane potential. Same method as in Figure 15. (After Frankenhaeuser and Hodgkin, 1957.)

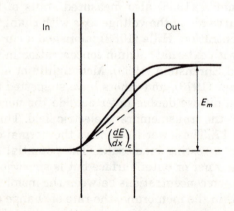

17

Schema to explain action of calcium on nerve membrane. Lower curve: Normal distribution of potential across membrane. Upper curve: Potential distribution with elevated external calcium concentration. $(dE/dx)_c$: Critical gradient for excitation. E_m: Measured transmembrane potential.

tial, is shown by the dotted line. Normally depolarization, or reduction of E_m, lowers the gradient to this level and results in excitation. When the external calcium concentration is increased above normal, a layer of Ca^{2+} ions forms near the surface of the membrane, loosely attracted by negative charges on the surface. This has the effect shown by the upper line: It makes the potential close to the outside surface more positive than normal, sharpening the corner of the potential curve. This change in the potential distribution can increase the transmembrane field strength without affecting E_m. Thus, with elevated external calcium a greater-than-normal depolarization is required to reduce the field in the membrane to the critical level. While somewhat speculative, this type of model is useful in combining many of the observations of Ca^{2+} action on nerve membranes, such as the lack of effect on resting potential and strong action on threshold.

More will be made of the use of calcium as an inward-current carrier by some cells, and of the regulation of intracellular Ca^{2+} concentration, in Chapter 8.

PROBLEMS

1. Using the data of Figure 3, plot membrane current at 0.5 msec after the start of the command pulse as ordinate (outward current is upward) versus potential to which the membrane is stepped (depolarizations to the right). On the same graph, plot the currents measured at 8 msec after the start of the pulse. At what potential does the early inward current pass through zero and become outward?

2. Using the normal data in Figure 5 and the same current and voltage conventions as in Problem 1, plot the currents at 0.5 and 5.5 msec after the start of the stimulus versus membrane potential. On the same graph plot the corresponding currents in Na^+-free solution. Does replacement of external sodium affect the late outward current?

3. For a depolarization to -4 mV, measure and tabulate the currents in Figure 5 in normal and Na^+-free solutions versus time, using 0.25-msec intervals. From these data, plot I_{Na} and I_K versus time on the same graph.

4. In Problem 3, E_{Na} was $+60$ mV and E_K was -70 mV. Calculate g_{Na} and g_K (in mS/cm^2) versus time, and plot. What is the peak value of g_{Na}? The final value of g_K?

REFERENCES

Adelman, W. J., Dyro, F. M., and Senft, J. 1965. Long duration responses obtained from internally perfused axons. *J. Gen. Physiol.* 48, 1–9.

Adelman, W. J., and Gilbert, D. L. 1964. Internally perfused squid axons studied under voltage clamp conditions. *J. Cell. Comp. Physiol.* 64, 423–428.

Armstrong, C. M., and Binstock, L. 1965. Anomalous rectification in the squid giant axon injected with tetraethylammonium chloride. *J. Gen. Physiol.* 48, 859–872.

Baker, P. F., Hodgkin, A. L., and Shaw, T. I. 1961. Replacement of the protoplasm of a giant nerve fibre with artificial solutions. *Nature (Lond.)* 190, 885–887.

Blaustein, M. P., and Goldman, D. E. 1966. Competitive action of calcium and procaine on lobster axon. *J. Gen. Physiol.* 49, 1043–1063.

Brismar, T. 1973. Effects of ionic concentration on permeability properties of nodal membranes in myelinated nerve fibres of *Xenopus laevis*; potential clamp experiments. *Acta Physiol. Scand.* 87, 474–484.

Cole, K. S. 1949. Dynamic electrical characteristics of the squid axon membrane. *Arch. Sci. Physiol.* 3, 253–258.

D'Arrigo, J. S. 1973. Possible screening of surface charges on crayfish axons by polyvalent metal ions. *J. Physiol.* 231, 117–128.

Frankenhaeuser, B. 1960. Quantitative description of sodium currents in myelinated nerve fibres of *Xenopus laevis*. *J. Physiol.* 151, 491–501.

Frankenhaeuser, B. 1963. A quantitative description of potassium currents in myelinated nerve fibres of *Xenopus laevis*. *J. Physiol.* 169, 424–430.

Frankenhaeuser, B., and Hodgkin, A. L. 1957. The action of calcium on the electrical properties of squid axons. *J. Physiol.* 137, 218–244.

Gilbert, D. L., and Ehrenstein, G. 1969. Effect of divalent cations on potassium conductance of squid axons: determination of surface charge. *Biophys. J.* 9, 447–463.

Hille, B. 1968. Charges and potentials at the nerve surface. Divalent ions and pH. *J. Gen. Physiol.* 51, 221–236.

Hodgkin, A. L., and Huxley, A. F. 1952a. Currents carried by sodium and potassium ions through the membrane of the giant axon of *Loligo*. *J. Physiol.* 116, 449–472.

Hodgkin, A. L., and Huxley, A. F. 1952b. The components of membrane conductance in the giant axon of *Loligo*. *J. Physiol.* 116, 473–496.

Hodgkin, A. L., and Huxley, A. F. 1952c. The dual effect of membrane potential on sodium conductance in the giant axon of *Loligo*. *J. Physiol.* 116, 497–506.

Hodgkin, A. L., Huxley, A. F., and Katz, B. 1952. Measurement of current-voltage relations in the membrane of the giant axon of *Loligo*. *J. Physiol.* 116, 424–448.

Hodgkin, A. L., and Katz, B. 1949. The effect of sodium ions on the electrical activity of the giant axon of the squid. *J. Physiol.* 108, 37–77.

Marmont, G. 1949. Studies on the axon membrane I. A new method. *J. Cell. Comp. Physiol.* 34, 351–382.

McLaughlin, S. G. A., Szabo, G., and Eisenman, G. 1971. Divalent ions and the surface potential of charged phospholipid membranes. *J. Gen. Physiol.* 58, 667–687.

Moore, J. W., Narahashi, T., and Ulbricht, W. 1963. Sodium conductance shift in an axon internally perfused with a low K solution. *Fed. Proc.* 22, 174.

Tasaki, I., and Singer, I. 1966. Membrane macromolecules and nerve excitability: a physico-chemical interpretation of excitation in squid giant axons. *Ann. N. Y. Acad. Sci.* 137, 792–806.

6

THE HODGKIN-HUXLEY MODEL
AND OTHER THEORIES
OF EXCITATION

PREDICTION OF VOLTAGE-CLAMP CURRENTS

It is important to note that there are really two parts to the HODGKIN-HUXLEY THEORY: (1) Their parallel-conductance model of the axon membrane, which, in conjunction with the voltage-clamp experiments, yielded so much valuable information, and (2) the mathematical model, which was constructed to describe the voltage and time dependencies of the conductances (Hodgkin and Huxley, 1952d). Other models have also attempted to account for the known properties of the Na^+ and K^+ currents, which are well established. The original Hodgkin-Huxley theory was intended to account for the following observations from the voltage-clamp experiments: (1) separate currents carried by Na^+ and K^+ ions (Hodgkin and Huxley, 1952a), (2) a potassium conductance that turns on with an S-shaped time course following a step depolarization (Hodgkin and Huxley, 1952b), and (3) a sodium conductance that turns on and then inactivates (Hodgkin and Huxley, 1952c).

The starting assumption for this theory is that there are separate currents carried by sodium, potassium, and other ions and that the transmembrane current in the voltage clamp is given by

$$I = C_m \frac{dE}{dt} + g_{Na}(E - E_{Na}) + g_K(E - E_K) + g_l(E - E_l) \tag{1}$$

where I = current density, A/cm^2
  E = membrane potential, V
  C_m = membrane capacity, F/cm^2
  g_{Na} = sodium conductance, S/cm^2
  g_K = potassium conductance, S/cm^2
  g_l = leak conductance, S/cm^2
  E_{Na} = sodium equilibrium potential, V
  E_K = potassium equilibrium potential, V
  E_l = leak equilibrium potential, V

This equation describes the current across an excitable structure whose interior is isopotential (no longitudinal spread of current). The conductances g_{Na} and g_K are assumed to vary in a deterministic way. The leak conductance is assumed constant. Under voltage-clamp conditions, the rate of change of potential is zero, and the membrane currents are purely ionic and should be given by the last three terms of Equation 1. In order to see if the model can predict real membrane currents, it is first necessary to write expressions for g_{Na} and g_K as functions of potential and time.

THEORETICAL POTASSIUM AND SODIUM CONDUCTANCES

The potassium conductance is described by

$$g_K = \bar{g}_K n^4 \tag{2}$$

where $\bar{g}_K$ = maximum potassium conductance, a constant
  n = a dimensionless variable that varies from 0 to 1 as a function of voltage and time

The fourth power of n is needed to describe the slow buildup of g_K following a step depolarization. The physical analogue of such a process is that four particles must be near the inside of the membrane at once in order for potassium ions to cross, where the probability of each particle being there is n. The differential equation governing n is

$$dn/dt = \alpha_n(1 - n) - \beta_n n \tag{3}$$

where α_n = rate constant for movement of particles from outside to inside, sec^{-1}
  β_n = rate constant for movement of particles from inside to outside, sec^{-1}

α_n and β_n are assumed to vary with voltage but not with time. If the particles are negatively charged, then α_n should increase and β_n

should decrease when the membrane is depolarized (that is, it should be easier to move the negative particles from the outside to the inside). The solution to Equation 3 when $n = n_0$ at $t = 0$ is

$$n = n_\infty - (n_\infty - n_0)e^{-t/\tau_n} \tag{4}$$

where $n_\infty = \alpha_n/(\alpha_n + \beta_n)$
$\tau_n = 1/(\alpha_n + \beta_n)$

n builds up exponentially with time following a depolarization, as shown in the top part of Figure 1, and n^4 follows the shape of the observed potassium conductance.

The sodium current is a little more complicated because it inactivates. In order to include this current in their theory, Hodgkin and Huxley assumed that

$$g_{Na} = \bar{g}_{Na}m^3h \tag{5}$$

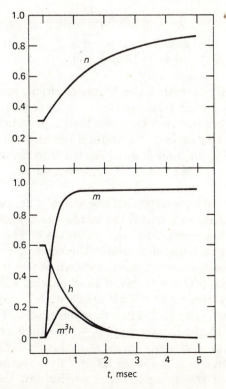

1 Variation of Hodgkin-Huxley parameters with time following a step depolarization in a voltage-clamped axon.

where $\bar{g}_{Na}$ = maximum sodium conductance, a constant

m = an activation parameter like n and that varies from 0 to 1 as a function of voltage and time

h = an inactivation parameter that varies from 0 to 1 as a function of voltage and time

The physical analogue of the activation and inactivation process is that three m particles must be near the inside of the membrane and an h particle must be on the outside (*not* on the inside—h particles are inactivating) for sodium ions to cross. The differential equations governing m and h are

$$dm/dt = \alpha_m(1 - m) - \beta_m \tag{6}$$

$$dh/dt = \alpha_h(1 - h) - \beta_h \tag{7}$$

where the rate constants are functions of voltage but not of time. The solutions, assuming $m = m_0$ and $h = h_0$ at $t = 0$, are

$$m = m_\infty - (m_\infty - m_0)e^{-t/\tau_m} \tag{8}$$

$$h = h_\infty - (h_\infty - h_0)e^{-t/\tau_h} \tag{9}$$

where $m_\infty = \alpha_m/(\alpha_m + \beta_m)$ and $\tau_m = 1/(\alpha_m + \beta_m)$
$h_\infty = \alpha_h/(\alpha_h + \beta_h)$ and $\tau_h = 1/(\alpha_h + \beta_h)$

m builds up exponentially with a short time constant, and h falls off exponentially with a longer time constant, as shown in the bottom part of Figure 1. The product m^3h then has the shape indicated, which corresponds to the time course of the sodium conductance. When the theoretical values of n, m, and h are inserted into Equation 1, the predicted currents are quite close to those measured with the voltage clamp.

In addition, the theory could predict the shape of action potentials in the length-clamped axon (in which the inside was made isopotential by means of a metal electrode). To do this, Hodgkin and Huxley solved Equation 1 by numerical methods under the condition that E was allowed to vary. Three such solutions are shown at the top of Figure 2. The "theoretical" axon was first given short shocks, whose intensities are indicated by the numbers alongside each trace. Then the membrane potential was calculated as a function of time. The smallest stimulus produced a slight depolarization, which then decayed back to the resting potential. A slightly larger stimulus finally gave rise to a spike, which reached a height of over 100 mV from resting. Stronger depolarizations caused the spike to occur earlier, but the overshoot was relatively constant. The bottom of Figure 2 shows some action

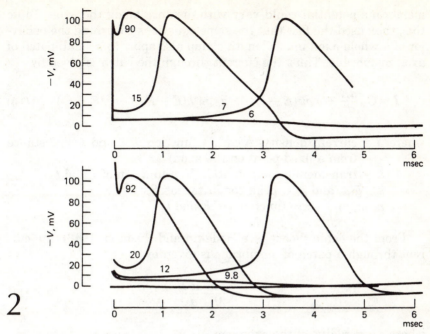

2

Calculated and observed action potentials in length-clamped axon. Top: Theoretical action potentials following short stocks to the axon. Bottom: Measured action potentials following similar stimulation of real axon. (From Hodgkin and Huxley, 1952c.)

potentials from real axons, for comparison with the model results. The predictions are fairly close quantitatively, as well as in form. (It should be noted that these curves were obtained for an axon at 6°C, much colder than the normal ocean temperature at which the squid live [perhaps 12 to 18°C]. Hodgkin and Huxley used low temperatures to slow the axon responses as an aid to obtaining a good voltage clamp. The theoretical values of n, m, and h would have to have much shorter time constants at higher ambient temperatures.)

PREDICTION OF PROPAGATED ACTION POTENTIAL

The above theoretical conductances were calculated for length-clamped axons that responded with the same transmembrane potential in all active areas. However, Hodgkin and Huxley were able to apply their theory to axons that were not length-clamped, where the membrane potential could vary with distance along the axon. To do this, they used the fact that the same equations governing the behavior of a whole axon under length clamp also apply to a small patch of axon membrane. Thus, the current through the patch is given by

$$I = C_m \frac{dE}{dt} + \bar{g}_K n^4 (E - E_K) + \bar{g}_{Na} m^3 h (E - E_{Na}) + \bar{g}_l (E - E_l) \qquad (10)$$

where I = current density, A/cm^2, a function of x and t (x, distance from a fixed point on the axon)
  E = transmembrane potential, V, a function of x and t
  $\bar{g}_K$, $\bar{g}_{Na}$, and $\bar{g}_l$ = peak conductances, S/cm^2
  n, m, and h are functions of E and t.

From the cable theory (see Hodgkin and Rushton, 1946), the current through a patch of membrane is given by

$$I = \frac{a}{2R_a} \frac{d^2E}{dx^2} \qquad (11)$$

where a = radius of the axon, cm
  R_a = specific resistivity of the axoplasm, ohm·cm

From Equations 10 and 11, it is possible to write a partial differential equation for E at any point on the axon. However, E is expressed in terms of t in Equation 10 and in terms of x in Equation 11, which makes the solution very difficult. A trick can now be used to circumvent this problem: Because the action potential is known to be propagated with a constant velocity, it may be expressed as

$$E = f(x - \theta t) \qquad (12)$$

where θ = conduction velocity, m/sec. This is an expression for a traveling wave, and it has the property that if the potential at time x has a certain time course, the potential at a point θt away from x will have the *same* time course as that at x, but delayed by t. Now, if we let $w = x - \theta t$, we can find the spatial derivative $\delta^2 E/\delta x^2$ in terms of the time derivative $\delta^2 E/\delta t^2$ (Slater and Frank, 1947):

$$\frac{\delta E}{\delta x} = \frac{\delta E}{\delta w} \qquad (13)$$

$$\frac{\delta^2 E}{\delta x^2} = \frac{\delta^2 E}{\delta w^2} \qquad (14)$$

$$\frac{\delta E}{\delta t} = -\theta \frac{\delta E}{\delta w} \tag{15}$$

$$\frac{\delta^2 E}{\delta t^2} = \theta^2 \frac{\delta^2 E}{\delta w^2} \tag{16}$$

From Equations 14 and 16,

$$\frac{\delta^2 E}{\delta x^2} = \frac{1}{\theta^2} \frac{\delta^2 E}{\delta t^2} \tag{17}$$

Equation 10 can now be written as a function of time only, using Equations 11 and 17:

$$\frac{a}{2R_a \theta^2} \frac{d^2 E}{dt^2} = C_m \frac{dE}{dt} + \bar{g}_K n^4 (E - E_K) + \bar{g}_{Na} m^3 h(E - E_{Na}) + \bar{g}_l(E - E_l) \tag{18}$$

The spatial variable x has now been removed from the potential equation. This is possible because all solutions for any x are the same functions of time, just delayed by an amount x/θ.

Equation 18 can now be solved by assuming values of the conduction velocity, θ, and using an iterative process. For most values of θ, the potential becomes infinite after an action potential. The correct value of θ is that for which the potential returns to resting after an impulse.

The behaviors of the sodium and potassium conductances can also be studied during the action potential, and are shown in Figure 3. V_{Na} and V_K are the sodium and potassium equilibrium potentials, and g_{Na} and g_K are the theoretical sodium and potassium conductances. V is the action potential calculated from Equation 18, where $V = E - E_r$ (E_r, resting potential). The propagated action potential is not substantially different from that in the length-clamped axon; both have about the same amplitude, and both exhibit an UNDERSHOOT, or hyperpolarization following the spike, to a level slightly more negative than resting.

THRESHOLD AND OTHER MEMBRANE PHENOMENA

The Hodgkin-Huxley equations could thus account for the time course of the propagated action potential in terms of the known variation of membrane conductances with potential and time. These equations could also explain some other membrane phenomena, including the threshold, or critical depolarization, for production of the action po-

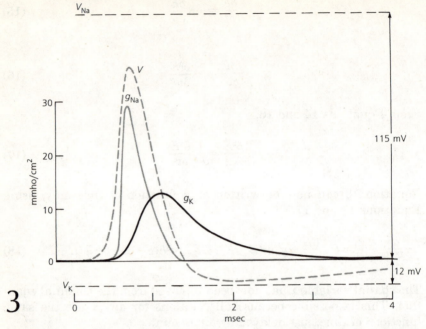

3

Theoretical changes in sodium and potassium conductances and membrane potential during a propagated nerve impulse. (From Hodgkin, 1964.)

tential. Because the sodium conductance is increased transiently by depolarization and because increased g_{Na} in turn leads to further depolarization, the change in membrane potential during a spike is *regenerative*. This may be schematized as

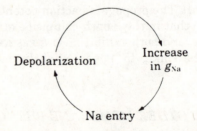

The slower-rising potassium conductance has the opposite effect, namely, to hyperpolarize the membrane.

The THRESHOLD potential may be defined as that potential at which the inward Na^+ current is just equal to the outward K^+ current. If the K^+ current is larger, the potential will return to resting. If the Na^+ current is larger, the potential will become unstable and produce a spike.

Furthermore, the Hodgkin-Huxley mathematical model could account for REFRACTORINESS, or the decreased excitability of an axon following an action potential. Two factors contributed to this property: (1) the fact the g_{Na} was somewhat inactivated following a spike and so could not reach as large a value in response to a second stimulus and (2) the persistence of the potassium conductance following a spike (see Figure 3). The amount of g_K that remains activated gives rise to the after-hyperpolarization, or undershoot, of the action potential and also makes it more difficult to achieve a sodium current that exceeds the potassium current. The time course of the refractory period in the squid axon is quite similar to those of g_K and h, the Na inactivation parameter (Hodgkin and Huxley, 1952d). Thus, the refractory period may be understood in terms of known potential and time variations of the conductances.

Other membrane phenomena that the Hodgkin-Huxley equations can explain include ANODE-BREAK EXCITATION and ACCOMMODATION. "Anode-break" refers to the removal of a hyperpolarizing stimulus, which, in the squid axon and other nerve membranes, often gives rise to an action potential. This is predicted from the removal of resting Na inactivation by the hyperpolarizing pulse (see Chapter 5). Accommodation is most often used to mean an increase in threshold with decreasing rate of rise of a stimulus (see, for example, Araki and Otani, 1959; and Bradley and Somjen, 1961). Occasionally it is used to mean slowing of repetitive discharge during a maintained stimulus. In either case, it is simply explained by Na inactivation and K activation during a depolarizing stimulus.

The success of the Hodgkin-Huxley equations in predicting these and other membrane phenomena showed the utility of mathematical modeling of this type. Even though the time and voltage dependencies of the conductances were known from experiment, it was not obvious that they would work together in concert to predict the action potential, threshold, refractoriness, and accommodation. The model showed that they could do so.

CONFIRMATION OF PREDICTED ION MOVEMENTS

Further verification of the ionic theory was provided by measurements of actual ion fluxes using radioisotopes. In 1951, Keynes showed that the extra net sodium influx during stimulation of cephalopod axons was about 4 pmol/cm^2/impulse. Calculation of the net Na^+ influx from the Hodgkin-Huxley equations gave approximately the same result.

An even more convincing demonstration of the sodium influx during activity was provided by Atwater et al. (1969), who measured it *during* a voltage-clamp experiment on an internally perfused squid axon. They were able to show that the measured sodium influx per impulse was at least 0.92 times the computed ionic flux and that the potential at which the measured ionic flux disappeared was the same as the reversal potential for the early inward current.

The accumulation of potassium ions outside an active muscle fiber has been measured directly with K^+-sensitive electrodes (Hník et al., 1972). The same measurement has been performed with snail neurons by Neher and Lux (1972, 1973). In these cells, the excess amount of potassium around the outside following a voltage-clamp pulse is approximately equal to that carried by the outward clamp current. All of these and more recent experiments make it difficult not to accept the idea that an action potential results from an early inward current that is carried by sodium, and a later outward current that is carried by potassium.

MODIFICATION OF THE MODEL FOR THE NODE OF RANVIER

The behavior of single Ranvier nodes under voltage-clamp conditions is best described by a slightly different formulation than that given by Hodgkin and Huxley for the squid axon. Frankenhaeuser (1960, 1963) found that the instantaneous *I-V* relations for sodium and potassium in single Ranvier nodes were not linear (as in Figures 7 and 8, Chapter 5). This meant that Equations 1 and 2, Chapter 5, could not be used to describe the Na^+ and K^+ currents. Instead, Frankenhaeuser used expressions for the currents derived from the constant-field theory (Hodgkin and Katz, 1949):

$$I_{Na} = P_{Na} \frac{F^2 E}{RT} \frac{[Na]_o - [Na]_i \exp{(EF/RT)}}{1 - \exp{(EF/RT)}} \tag{19}$$

$$I_K = P_K \frac{F^2 E}{RT} \frac{[K]_o - [K]_i \exp{(EF/RT)}}{1 - \exp{(EF/RT)}} \tag{20}$$

where P = permeability
F = Faraday constant
E = membrane potential
R = universal gas constant
T = temperature, K

To describe the kinetics of the sodium and potassium currents, Frankenhaeuser used the forms

$$P_{Na} = \bar{P}_{Na} m^2 h \tag{21}$$

$$P_K = \bar{P}_K n^2 k \tag{22}$$

where m and h have the same meanings as in the Hodgkin-Huxley model

n is a potassium activation parameter, as in the Hodgkin-Huxley model

k is a slow inactivation parameter for the potassium current.

Other than the m^2 dependence for the sodium current and the potassium inactivation factor, the behavior of the single node was well described by this version of the Hodgkin-Huxley theory.

ALTERNATIVE MODELS

While the mathematical model of Hodgkin and Huxley predicts the ionic currents in the squid axon quite well, it is not the only model that can do this. Another approach was that of Hoyt (1963), who used empirical relationships for g_{Na} and g_K that were chosen to fit the observed currents exactly. For instance, g_K was assumed to be a function of v_K, a parameter like the Hodgkin-Huxley n, having the form

$$v_K = v_{K_\infty}(1 - e^{-\alpha_K t}) \tag{23}$$

where v_{K_∞} = final value of v_K
  α_K = inverse time constant

Then v_K was chosen to give the correct values of g_K at different potentials and times. It turned out that for small values of g_K the empirical relationship was

$$g_K = \bar{g}_K(v_K + C)^p \tag{24}$$

where $\bar{g}_K$ = maximum K conductance
  C = constant
  p = constant exponent

For larger values of g_K, the curve was less rapidly rising with v_K than in Equation 24. For the sodium channel, instead of assuming that g_{Na} depended on two parameters, such as m and h, she assumed that it varied with one parameter, v_{Na}, which had the form

$$v_{Na} = A(1 - e^{-at}) - B(1 - e^{-bt}) \tag{25}$$

ν_{Na} was chosen empirically to give the correct values of g_{Na} at different potentials and times.

This model can predict every behavior of the squid axon that is predicted by the Hodgkin-Huxley equations. It gives better fits to the g_{Na} and g_K curves, because it is constructed empirically from those conductances. In addition, Hoyt's model can account for the very slow rise of K^+ current following a strong hyperpolarization (see Chapter 7), which is not a feature of the original Hodgkin-Huxley theory.

Goldman (1964) took a very different approach from that of Hodgkin and Huxley; he assumed that the ion carriers in the membrane are the same for sodium as for potassium. The carriers are thought to have binding sites that can exchange Na^+ for K^+ and also Ca^{2+}. This is outlined as shown:

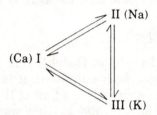

The sites may be in any of three states: In state I, the resting condition, the sites preferentially bind calcium. Depolarization causes many of the sites to pass into state II, and bind sodium. This is the state that gives rise to the early inward current in the voltage clamp. In state III the sites bind potassium, and this produces the late outward current. Finally, the sites return to state I. It is assumed that there are n_{Na} sites per square centimeter in the Na state, n_K in the K state, and n_{Ca} in the Ca state, at any time. Goldman calculated the potential and time dependence of the n's, and from this the variation of n_{Na} and n_K following a step depolarization. These are shown in Figure 4. While no quantitative comparison was made to Hodgkin and Huxley's experimental data, the similarity to the curves of g_{Na} and g_K in the voltage-clamped squid axon is striking.

In both of these alternative models, different approaches from that of Hodgkin and Huxley were used to predict the same voltage-clamp currents. These currents are a permanent fact about squid axon membranes and will always have to be explained by new theories. Perhaps because of priority, the Hodgkin-Huxley theory has dominated the study of excitation since it appeared. However, many other mechanisms have been proposed to replace the movement of n, m, and h particles. These include ion induction (Ling, 1962), ion exchange (Tasaki, 1968), storage of sodium in the area of the membrane (Hoyt and

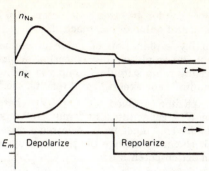

4

Variation of number of sodium-binding (n_{Na}) and potassium-binding (n_K) sites per square centimeter with time following a depolarization. Follows Goldman's theory of excitation (1964). E_m: membrane potential.

Strieb, 1971), flipping of dipoles in the membrane (Wei, 1972), and more generally, a movement of ions past a series of energy barriers in the membrane (Hille, 1975). These models are mentioned to illustrate the range of hypotheses that have been proposed to explain excitation. Nowadays, most if not all excitable systems have been shown to involve the opening and closing of ION CHANNELS in the membrane, which will be covered extensively in Chapters 11–13.

PROBLEMS

1. After a particular step depolarization in Hodgkin and Huxley's model axon, the parameters of the potassium conductance are

$$n_\infty = 0.891$$
$$n_0 = 0.315$$
$$\tau_n = 1.70 \text{ msec}$$
$$\bar{g}_K = 24.3 \text{ mS/cm}^2$$

Plot g_K as a function of time for 10 msec, using steps of 0.5 msec for the fast-rising part (up to 4 msec). What is the final value of g_K?

2. After the same depolarization as in Problem 1, the parameters of the sodium conductance are

$$m_\infty = 0.963$$
$$m_0 = 0$$
$$\tau_m = 0.252 \text{ msec}$$
$$h_\infty = 0$$
$$h_0 = 0.605$$
$$\tau_h = 0.840 \text{ msec}$$
$$\bar{g}_{Na} = 70.7 \text{ mS/cm}^2$$

Plot g_{Na} as a function of time for 10 msec, using steps of 0.2 msec for up to 2 msec. What is the largest value of g_{Na} reached?

3. From the Hodgkin-Huxley explanation of nerve accommodation, what would you predict about the amplitude (overshoot) of an action potential produced by a slowly rising ramp stimulus, compared with that produced by a rapidly rising stimulus? (For experimental results, see Vallbö, 1964).

4. The charge across a capacitor is given by $q = CV$, where q = charge separation in coulombs, C = capacitance in farads, and V = potential in volts. How many coulombs/cm^2 must be transferred across a membrane with a capacitance of 1 μF/cm^2 to change the potential by 100 mV (about the same amount as an action potential)?

5. Since there is one faraday (96,500 coulombs) in a mole of charged particles, how many mol/cm^2 had to cross the membrane in Problem 4 to change the potential by 100 mV? Can you account for any discrepancy between the answer to this problem and the amount of charge found by Keynes for net sodium entry during an action potential?

6. After a step depolarization in the Hoyt model of the squid axon, the sodium parameter, v_{Na}, follows the curve

$$v_{Na} = 71.0(1 - e^{-t/0.219}) - 53.7(1 - e^{-t/1.20})$$

g_{Na} varies monotonically with v_{Na}. Plot the time course of v_{Na} for the first 10 msec after the start of the depolarization. What is the largest value of v_{Na} reached?

REFERENCES

Araki, T., and Otani, T. 1959. Accommodation and local response in motoneurones of toad's spinal cord. *Jpn. J. Physiol.* 9, 69–83.

Atwater, I., Bezanilla, F., and Rojas, E. 1969. Sodium influxes in internally perfused squid giant axon during voltage clamp. *J. Physiol.* 201, 657–664.

Bradley, K., and Somjen, G. G. 1961. Accommodation in motoneurones of the rat and cat. *J. Physiol.* 156, 75–92.

Frankenhaeuser, B. 1960. Quantitative description of sodium currents in myelinated nerve fibres of *Xenopus laevis*. *J. Physiol.* 151, 491–501.

Frankenhaeuser, B. 1963. A quantitative description of potassium currents in myelinated nerve fibres of *Xenopus laevis*. *J. Physiol.* 169, 424–430.

Goldman, D. E. 1964. A molecular structural basis for the excitation properties of axons. *Biophys. J.* 4, 167–188.

Hille, B. 1975. Ionic selectivity, saturation, and block in sodium channels: a four-barrier model. *J. Gen. Physiol.* 66, 535–560.

Hník, P., Vyskočil, F., Kříž, N., and Holas, M. 1972. Work-induced increase of extracellular potassium concentration in muscle measured by ion-specific electrodes. *Brain Res.* 40, 559–562.

Hodgkin, A. L. 1964. *The Conduction of the Nervous Impulse*. Springfield, Ill., Thomas, p. 63.

Hodgkin, A. L., and Huxley, A. F. 1952a. Currents carried by sodium and potassium ions through the membrane of the giant axon of *Loligo*. *J. Physiol.* 116, 449–472.

Hodgkin, A. L., and Huxley, A. F. 1952b. The components of membrane conductance in the giant axon of *Loligo*. *J. Physiol.* 116, 473–496.

Hodgkin, A. L., and Huxley, A. F. 1952c. The dual effect of membrane potential on sodium conductance in the giant axon of *Loligo*. *J. Physiol.* 116, 497–506.

Hodgkin, A. L., and Huxley, A. F. 1952d. A quantitative description of membrane current and its application to conduction and excitation in nerve. *J. Physiol.* 117, 500–544.

Hodgkin, A. L., and Katz, B. 1949. The effect of sodium ions on the electrical activity of the giant axon of the squid. *J. Physiol.* 108, 37–77.

Hodgkin, A. L., and Rushton, W. A. H. 1946. The electrical constants of a crustacean nerve fibre. *Proc. R. Soc. B.* 133, 444–479.

Hoyt, R. C. 1963. The squid giant axon: mathematical models. *Biophys. J.* 3, 399–431.

Hoyt, R., and Strieb, J. D. 1971. A stored charge model for the sodium channel. *Biophys. J.* 11, 868–885.

Keynes, R. D. 1951. The ionic movements during nervous activity. *J. Physiol.* 114, 119–150.

Ling, G. 1962. *A Physical Theory of the Living State: The Association-Induction Hypothesis.* New York, Blaisdell.

Neher, E., and Lux, H. D. 1972. Messung extrazellulärer K-Anreicherung während eines Voltage-Clamp-Pulses. *Pflügers Arch. Eur. J. Physiol.* 336, 87.

Neher, E., and Lux, H. D. 1973. Rapid changes of potassium concentration at the outer surface of exposed single neurons during membrane current flow. *J. Gen. Physiol.* 61, 385–399.

Slater, J. C., and Frank, N. H. 1947. *Mechanics.* New York, McGraw-Hill, p. 163.

Tasaki, I. 1968. *Nerve Excitation: A Macromolecular Approach.* Springfield, Ill., Thomas.

Vallbö, A. B. 1964. Accommodation related to inactivation of the sodium permeability in single myelinated nerve fibres from *Xenopus laevis*. *Acta Physiol. Scand.* 61, 429–444.

Wei, L. Y. 1972. Dipole theory of heat production and absorption in nerve axon. *Biophys. J.* 12, 1159–1170.

7

FURTHER STUDIES OF THE SODIUM
AND POTASSIUM CURRENTS

Many new discoveries concerning the behavior of membrane currents have been made since the time of Hodgkin and Huxley. Ionic selectivities have been determined for the inward and outward currents; specific blocking agents have been found for the Na^+ and K^+ channels; and sodium inactivation has been chemically removed in the squid axon, to name a few. Most exciting of all, the development of the tightly sealed PATCH PIPETTE (Chapter 11) has permitted recording the activity of one or a few single ion channels in restricted areas of membranes. These studies have shown that the active conductances are made up of *quantized*, or irreducible, subunits, due to the opening and closing of single channels. The total conductance is the sum over time of billions of these events per square centimeter. The single-channel conductance may be calculated from the binding of specific blocking compounds to channels, through measurement of net gating charge movement during a depolarization (this chapter), from spectral density functions of membrane current noise, and directly with the patch pipette technique (Chapters 11 and 12).

It is becoming increasingly clear that excitability is derived from more than just inward Na^+ and delayed outward K^+ currents: Some potassium currents have been discovered that have a transient (inactivating) time-course, unlike the delayed-current channels, and other K^+ currents have been found to be activated by an increase in intracellular calcium concentration. Calcium itself may serve as the inward current carrier for excitation (see Chapter 8). Many different neurotransmitters besides acetylcholine are known to activate membrane ionic channels (Chapter 10). These observations have all added to our understanding of how the many different types of ion channels participate in excitation. In this chapter we shall concentrate on the voltage, ion, and drug sensitivities of the different Na^+ and K^+ currents.

INDEPENDENT EFFECTS OF POTENTIAL ON SODIUM AND POTASSIUM CURRENTS

It is now clear that substantive differences exist between the mechanisms for sodium inflow and potassium outflow during the action potential. However, this was not always thought to be the case; some authors have argued that the same molecular machinery carries both the sodium and potassium currents (Mullins, 1959; Goldman, 1964; Tasaki, 1968). Such "coupled" models are at odds with the observations of this and the next two sections.

It is possible to alter the magnitude and time course of the sodium and potassium currents in voltage-clamped axons by conditioning depolarization or hyperpolarization. The effect of predepolarization is to inactivate the inward current without affecting the outward current (see Figures 9 to 13, Chapter 5). Cole and Moore (1960) showed that large conditioning hyperpolarizations (up to −212 mV absolute membrane potential) delay the onset of the outward current with little or no effect on the inward current. These outward currents, obtained from a two-step voltage clamp, are shown in Figure 1. First, the membrane was clamped for 3 msec to a potential between −52 and −212 mV; then it was depolarized to +60 mV (near the sodium equilibrium potential). The larger the prehyperpolarization, the greater was the delay of the potassium currents. In order to account for this delay, Cole and Moore found that it was necessary to use an expression of the form

$$I_K = \bar{g}_K n^{25}(E - E_K) \qquad (1)$$

instead of the fourth-power dependency used by Hodgkin and Huxley (cf. Equation 2, Chapter 6). The independent variability of the inward and outward currents in this example suggests that they are carried by separate mechanisms.

DIFFERENT ION SELECTIVITIES OF EARLY AND LATE CURRENTS

Different ion selectivities may be inferred by changing external ion concentrations around active neurons under voltage clamp and looking

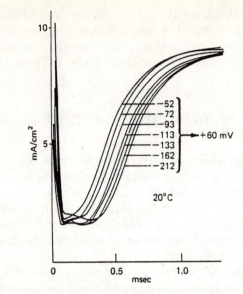

1

Effect of prehyperpolarization on outward currents in voltage-clamped squid axon. (From Cole and Moore, 1960.)

at the effects on early and late currents. As shown by Moore et al. (1966), the early inward current mechanism in the squid admits sodium and lithium but excludes potassium and rubidium. The late outward current mechanism admits potassium and rubidium but excludes sodium and lithium. The same relationships are seen in the node of Ranvier (Hille, 1972). Hence, it appears there are two separate mechanisms for the early and late currents, with completely different selectivities.

PHARMACOLOGICAL SPECIFICITIES OF THE EARLY AND LATE CURRENTS

Strong support for the idea of separate mechanisms came from the fortuitous discovery of agents that specifically block one current without affecting the other. In 1959, Hagiwara and Saito examined the effects of tetraethylammonium (TEA) on a voltage-clamped neuron. TEA has the following structure:

$$C_2H_5-\overset{\overset{\displaystyle C_2H_5}{|}}{\underset{\underset{\displaystyle C_2H_5}{|}}{N^+}}-C_2H_5$$

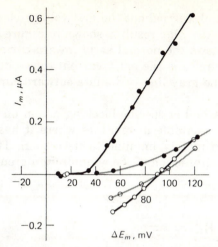

2

Effect of tetraethylammonium ion on outward currents in *Onchidium* neuron. I_m: Voltage clamp currents, ΔE_m: Membrane potential measured from resting. Open circles show early currents, solid dots late currents. Solid lines obtained in normal saline, gray lines in saline containing about 90-mM TEA. (From Hagiwara and Saito, 1959.)

Some of the results are shown in Figure 2. The open circles show the early inward current and the solid dots the late outward current. Application of TEA (gray lines) greatly reduced the outward current but had little effect on the inward current. This differential action has also been demonstrated in the squid axon (Armstrong and Binstock, 1965). In the node of Ranvier, the only Hodgkin-Huxley parameter affected by TEA is $\bar{g}_K$, the maximum potassium conductance (Hille, 1967). The effect of this compound on unclamped neurons is to prolong the action potential by greatly delaying and inhibiting the active repolarization.

Tetrodotoxin (TTX) is a neuroactive poison from the puffer fish; it has a specific blocking action on the early inward current (as does the related compound, saxitoxin, found in some salamanders). The TTX molecule has the following structure:

In 1965 Nakamura et al. carried out the first voltage-clamp study of TTX using the squid axon. One result is shown in Figure 3. The solid line with solid dots shows the normal early inward current, and the solid line with open circles is the early current (now outward) after application of TTX. The gray line is the late outward current, which is unaffected by TTX.

Tetrodotoxin has a highly specific blocking action on the sodium channel in almost all excitable membranes where it has been tried (the puffer fish is fortunately immune to its action). The blocking action may be due to interaction of the guanidinium group

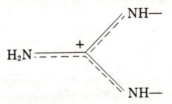

with the membrane Na^+ channels. The TTX molecule binds to the Na^+-selective channel but is too big to pass through the channel. The selective actions of TTX and TEA on nerve and muscle membranes thus imply that the compounds are acting on separate Na^+ and K^+ channels. (The possibility that both inward and outward currents were carried by the same channels was really laid to rest by the single-channel studies described in Chapter 11.)

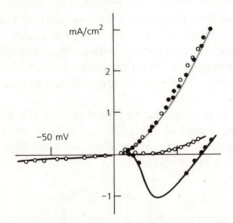

3

Effect of tetrodotoxin on inward currents in squid axon. Solid lines show early currents, gray line late currents. Solid dots were obtained in normal saline, open circles in saline containing 5×10^{-7} g/ml TTX. (From Nakamura et al., 1965.)

Agents or "probes" such as TTX that bind tightly to channels have also been used in the isolation and purification of these structures (Chapter 13).

DENSITY OF TTX BINDING SITES IN THE MEMBRANE

The binding of tetrodotoxin to nerve may also be used to estimate the number of sodium channels per unit area. This was first done with unlabeled TTX by Moore et al. (1967) and was subsequently refined with the use of tritiated TTX (Colquhoun et al., 1972; Hafemann, 1972). In these experiments, the nerve is soaked in a solution containing labeled TTX of a concentration just sufficient to block the action potentials. The amount of TTX taken up per gram of nerve tissue is then obtained by scintillation counting. From light and electron micrographs, the area of nerve membrane per gram of tissue is estimated. Assuming that one Na^+ channel is blocked by one molecule of TTX, it is then possible to estimate the channel density by dividing the TTX uptake by the area. By this method, Levinson and Meves (1975) calculated the channel density in the squid axon as $553 \pm 119/\mu m^2$ (mean $\pm$ SD), and Ritchie and Rogart (1977) found a density for the single node of Ranvier of $12,000/\mu m^2$.

The single-channel conductance may be calculated from this approach as

$$\gamma = \frac{\bar{g}_{Na}}{D} \qquad (2)$$

where γ = single-channel conductance, pS
   $\bar{g}_{Na}$ = peak sodium conductance, $pS/\mu m^2$
   D = channel density/μm^2

Hodgkin and Huxley (1952) estimated that $\bar{g}_{Na}$ for the squid axon was $1200\ pS/\mu m^2$, so γ is about 2.17 ± 0.5 pS. For the node of Ranvier, Nonner et al. (1975) found a $\bar{g}_{Na}$ of 15,000 to 20,000 $pS/\mu m^2$, so γ is 1.25 to 1.67 pS. Of course, there are many possible sources of error in this work, but the figures for the squid axon and node are interestingly close and agree with other methods of estimation (to be discussed).

REMOVAL OR SLOWING OF SODIUM INACTIVATION

For some years there was a dispute in the literature about whether activation and inactivation of the sodium current were coupled, i.e., whether a channel had to pass through an active form before it became inactivated. Two alternative models of a sodium channel during a positive voltage-clamp pulse are thus

I. Coupled: Sodium gate Closed → Open → Inactivated
II. Uncoupled: Activation gate Closed → Open
Inactivation gate Open → Closed

In Hodgkin and Huxley's (1952) model, the activation and inactivation processes were completely separate; no coupling was assumed between m and h. Some later models assumed a tight coupling of activation and inactivation (Mullins, 1959; Goldman, 1964). However, Hoyt (1963) showed that it is not necessary to describe g_{Na} by two first-order processes; a single variable that satisfies a second-order differential equation gives a good representation. Goldman (1975) pointed out that activation and inactivation may be part of the same process since they need not be separated mathematically.

Some direct pharmacological evidence was brought to bear on this issue by Armstrong et al. (1973). They found that in axons perfused for the correct length of time with the proteolytic enzyme mixture pronase, the sodium conductance did not inactivate. This is shown in Figure 4. The left side shows the voltage-clamp currents obtained in the presence of TEA, which are presumably carried by sodium. On the right side, after treatment of the axon with pronase, the sodium currents clearly do not inactivate. This indicates that the inactivation process is different from activation and lends considerable support to model II.

The component of pronase responsible for blocking inactivation has been identified as alkaline proteinase b (Rojas and Rudy, 1976), an

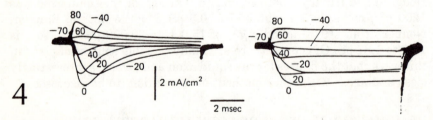

4

Destruction of Na^+ inactivation by perfusion of squid axon with pronase. Left: Voltage-clamp currents with 15-mM TEA in internal perfusate. Right: Same conditions after a 6-min perfusion with pronase. (From Armstrong et al., 1973.)

enzyme that cleaves at the carboxyl group of lysine and arginine residues. Eaton et al. (1978) applied three arginine-specific reagents inside squid axons and also removed inactivation, which strongly implicated arginine residues as the inactivation gates.

BLOCKAGE OF CURRENTS BY LOCAL ANESTHETICS

Taylor, in 1959, showed that the local anesthetic procaine blocked conduction and excitation in the squid axon by blocking the sodium current and reducing the potassium current. The subsequent studies with nodes of Ranvier (Strichartz, 1973; Hille et al., 1975) showed that this block was *use-dependent*, that is, it increased with increasing stimulation of the nerve fibers. This effect is shown in Figure 5. The single node is bathed in 0.5 mM lidocaine, and then 7-msec depolarizing pulses to -20 mV are applied at different frequencies. The sodium permeability (related to the inward Na$^+$ current) is indicated by the dots. At a frequency of 1/sec, the value of P_{Na} is little reduced from the normalized control value of 1. When the frequency of stimulation is increased to 2, 4, and 8/sec, the permeability steadily decreases. The anesthetic has a much stronger blocking action when the

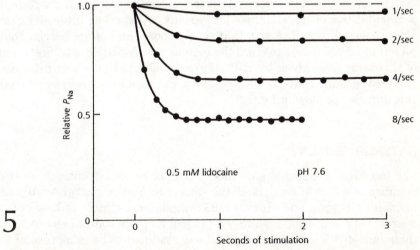

5

Use-dependent block of open Na channels by local anesthetic. 0.5 mM lidocaine placed around single node of Ranvier five min before start of stimulation. Top trace: Sodium permeability decreases slightly with repeated 1/sec stimuli. Lower traces: Faster rates of stimulation enhance anesthetic block. (From Hille et al., 1975.)

sodium channels have recently been stimulated, that is, when they are still open. This phenomenon is thus called OPEN-CHANNEL BLOCK or sometimes, USE-DEPENDENT BLOCK, meaning the more the channel has been used, the more it is blocked by the local anesthetic. This is usually interpreted to mean that the blocking site is somewhere inside the channel (Strichartz, 1973; Hille et al., 1975).

GATES AND FILTERS

In order to think about the mechanisms of the conductance increases that occur during excitation (a further reductionism—see the Introduction), it has become useful to divide the process into a VOLTAGE-SENSITIVE GATE and a connected SELECTIVITY FILTER. These are loose conceptual terms and need not signify any specific structure in the membrane. The gate analogy was first used to describe the steep voltage-conductance relation found by Hodgkin and Huxley. The gates open under the influence of a change in membrane electric field, allowing sodium to flow inward along its electrochemical gradient. The resulting depolarization causes more and more gates to open. The m and h variables in Hodgkin and Huxley's (1952) theory are their version of the gate since they contain all the voltage sensitivity of the sodium channel.

The concept of the selectivity filter is used to explain the different permeabilities of the channels for various cations. The filter and gate are connected in such a way that each imposes an energy barrier that an ion must overcome to cross the membrane. A simple interpretation of this scheme is given by Hille (1978), where the gate and filter are chemical groups that are located along the membrane pores and that can impede the flow of ions.

GATING CURRENT

The most likely way the gate mechanism could detect changes in the membrane electric field is if the gate contains a charge or dipole moment. Hodgkin and Huxley (1952) made an estimate of how much charge must cross the membrane to open a single sodium channel. In their model the sodium conductance is assumed to be proportional to the fraction of some gating "particles" that are near the inside (axoplasmic side) of the membrane:

$$g_{Na} = \overline{g}_{Na}P_i \qquad \qquad (3)$$

$$P_i + P_o = 1 \qquad \qquad (4)$$

where P_i = fraction of particles on the inside
$\quad\quad P_o$ = fraction of particles on the outside

If the particles move independently in the membrane, they will be arranged according to Boltzmann's distribution:

$$\frac{P_i}{P_o} = e^{(w+z\epsilon E)/kT} \tag{5}$$

where w = work required for a particle to cross the membrane when
$\quad\quad\quad E = 0$
$\quad\quad z$ = number of charges on the gating molecule
$\quad\quad \epsilon$ = electronic charge
$\quad\quad E$ = membrane potential
$\quad kT$ = 25.7 mV at 20°C

Combining Equations 3–5, the sodium conductance is

$$g_{Na} = \bar{g}_{Na} \frac{e^{(w+z\epsilon E)/kT}}{1 + e^{(w+z\epsilon E)/kT}} \tag{6}$$

When E is large and negative so that $e^{(w + z\epsilon E)/kT)} \ll 1$, then

$$\bar{g}_{Na} \cong \bar{g}_{Na} e^{z\epsilon E/kT} \tag{7}$$

Hodgkin and Huxley showed that, at large negative potentials, when $g_{Na} \ll \bar{g}_{Na}$,

$$g_{Na} \propto e^{E/4} \tag{8}$$

So $z = 6$, or six charges must cross the membrane (or 12 go half-way, etc.) to open one sodium channel; or if a dipole is assumed to reverse, it must have three charges at each end.

The movement of this gating charge is outward for a depolarizing pulse, and it gives rise to a small outward current. However, this outward current is masked by the inward sodium current and the large outward current required to charge the membrane capacitance (see Figure 2, Chapter 5), which overlap the gating current. In order to remove the ionic currents, Armstrong and Bezanilla (1973) perfused squid axons with cesium fluoride, which does not pass through the outward K^+ channels, and used the impermeant cation Tris instead of Na^+ in the external solution. In addition, they often added TTX to the outside solution to block any residual current through the Na^+ channels. To eliminate the linear capacitive current, they averaged the responses to an equal number of positive and negative steps of potential from the negative holding level. The resultant average current is shown in Figure 6, Part A (from Armstrong and Bezanilla, 1974). The outward current shown is the result of a greater outward current produced by the depolarizing pulses than the inward current produced by the hyperpolarizing pulses; is sometimes known as an ASYMMETRY CURRENT. It is thought to be produced by movement of charges or dipoles under the influence of the outward-directed electric field in the membrane; this movement does not occur with an inward-directed field. Part B shows the time course of the sodium current with sodium and no TTX in the external solution and indicates that the gating current precedes the sodium current. Part C is the gating current after termination of a positive step, and part D is the sodium current "tail" at the same time; these have a very similar time course.

The fact that TTX does not block gating currents means that the gate is remote from the blocking site. However, some procedures do block both the gating current and the inward sodium current: (1) perfusion of the axon with a solution containing 10 mM ZnCl$_2$, (2) predepolarization of the axon by short pulses or maintained depolarization (Bezanilla and Armstrong, 1974), and (3) perfusion with a solution containing 30 mM glutaraldehyde (Meves, 1974). It is usually said that the gate lies toward the inside of the membrane, since it is

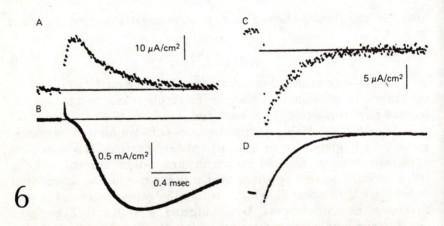

Gating currents in the squid, *Loligo*. A: Average difference in currents produced by 50 steps of potential from −70 to −140 mV and 50 steps from −70 to 0 mV. Axon blocked with external Na$^+$-free solution containing TTX and internal solution containing cesium. B: Inward sodium current in artificial seawater. C: Gating current after termination of pulses. D: Inward sodium current after termination of pulses. (From Armstrong and Bezanilla, 1974.)

only affected by internal perfusion, and that TTX blocks from the outside, since it is much more effective when applied externally (Armstrong, 1975).

The integral of the time course of gating current gives the net charge transferred during a single voltage clamp step. This can be as large as 1882 $\epsilon/\mu m^2$ (Keynes and Rojas, 1974). This charge, Q, should be related to the charge transferred per sodium gate, $z\epsilon$, by

$$Q = z\epsilon D \qquad (9)$$

where z has been estimated as six charges per gate
  ϵ = electronic charge
  D = density of gates/μm^2

Using the above value of Q, Equation 9 indicates a density of 314 gates/μm^2. Assuming one gate per channel, the single-channel conductance for the squid axon may be found from Equation 2 as 3.82 pS. Another way this data may be interpreted is to show that most or all of the asymmetry current measured by this technique is due to movement of gating molecules in the membrane: If the density of channels in the squid axon, from TTX-uptake experiments, is 553/μm^2, then the charge transfer predicted from Equation 9 is 3320 $\epsilon/\mu m^2$. Since the measured gating charge is only 1882 $\epsilon/\mu m^2$, there is scarcely enough to account for the theoretical movement of gating charge.

TRANSIENT OUTWARD CURRENT

Voltage-clamp studies with molluscan nerve cell bodies have revealed some potassium currents that are not described for the squid axon or node of Ranvier. These are the calcium-activated K^+ currents (which will be discussed in the next section), and the fast transient, or EARLY OUTWARD CURRENT. This was seen by Hagiwara et al. (1961) in *Onchidium* neurons and has been studied by Connor and Stevens (1971a) in nudibranchs and by Neher (1971) in snail neurons. An example is shown in Figure 7. The left side shows inward and outward currents resulting from a step depolarization from −48 to +5 mV. The center shows the response when the potential is held at −93 mV for 0.5 sec and then stepped to +5 mV. Presumably, the inward current in the center record is masked by a large transient outward current, which is inactivated at more positive holding potentials. The right side is a computer simulation: The down-then-up trace is a slightly magnified version of the currents on the left side of the figure. When it is subtracted from the total current shown in the center of the figure, the up-then-down curve of the transient current is seen by itself.

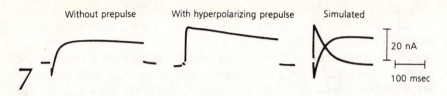

7

Transient outward current in *Helix* neuron. Left: Potential stepped from −48 to +5 mV. Center: Potential stepped from −93 to +5 mV. Right: Computer subtraction; up-then-down curve is difference between outward currents with and without hyperpolarizing prepulse. (From Neher, 1971.)

To describe this current, called I_A, or A-current, Connor and Stevens used the formula

$$I_A = K(1 - e^{-t/\tau_A})^N e^{-t/\tau_B} \tag{10}$$

where K = a constant
τ_A = rising time constant
τ_B = falling time constant
N = an empirically determined exponent

They also observed that the A-current is only reduced about 50% by concentrations of TEA that completely block the late voltage-sensitive K^+ current. Thompson (1977) showed that the compound 4-aminopyridine specifically blocks I_A without affecting the late voltage-sensitive current.

The significance of the fast transient current may be that it acts to slow membrane responses following a period of hyperpolarization. The undershoot of an action potential is sufficient to reduce the inactivation of I_A, and this current may permit the slow type of repetitive firing seen in these neurons (Connor and Stevens, 1971b; see Chapter 9). A-currents also have the distinction of being the first to be removed from a type of living membrane by mutagenesis, which led to the sequencing of the gene for the associated ion channels (Chapter 13).

Ca^{2+}-ACTIVATED POTASSIUM CURRENT

In 1970, Meech and Strumwasser first demonstrated that injection of calcium ions into nerve cells caused an increase in potassium conductance. This finding is illustrated in Figure 8 (from Meech, 1972).

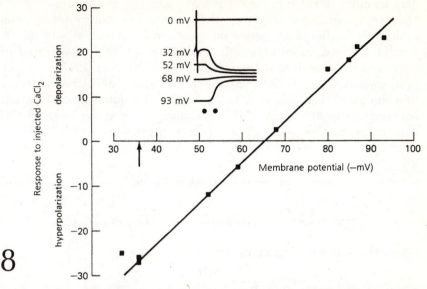

Calcium-activated potassium conductance in *Aplysia* neuron. Inset: Potential changes upon injection of small amounts of 3 *M* CaCl₂ between the dots. Potential held by applied current at levels shown, before Ca injection. Graph: reversal of direction of Ca response by varying initial holding potential. Arrow shows resting potential. (From Meech, 1972.)

The inset shows changes in membrane potential of an *Aplysia* neuron in response to small amounts of $CaCl_2$ injected during the period between the two dots (5 msec apart). By varying the initial potential with applied current, the direction of the Ca^{2+} response can be reversed. The graph shows the magnitude and sign of the response as a function of membrane potential before Ca^{2+} injection. The reversal potential, i.e., the membrane potential at which Ca^{2+} injection causes no response, varies with external potassium concentration; this shows that calcium is activating a membrane potassium conductance.

The importance of this work soon became evident since it could explain slow changes in potassium conductance following a burst of activity in neurons with a known inward calcium current (Brodwick and Junge, 1972). Removal of external calcium or injection of a Ca^{2+}-accumulating compound, ethylene glycol bis(β-amino-ethylether)-N,N'-tetraacetic acid (EGTA), abolished the post-burst hyperpolarization seen in *Aplysia* cells (Meech, 1974). In a study of *Helix* neurons, Meech and Standen (1975) distinguished between two kinds of potassium conductance: one was voltage sensitive and the other was dependent on entry of calcium ions. The Ca^{2+}-activated potassium conductance was much slower than the voltage-sensitive conductance and was selectively inhibited by magnesium ions in the external solution. A similar Ca^{2+}-activated potassium current was also demonstrated in crab muscle fibers at that time (Mounier and Vassort, 1975).

Brown et al. (1977) injected buffered solutions of calcium chloride into the giant (R2) cell in *Aplysia* and found a quantitative relation between the total membrane conductance, G_m, and the internal calcium concentration, $[Ca]_i$. This may be expressed as

$$\frac{G_m}{G_m^0} = 1; \quad [Ca]_i < 10^{-7} M$$

$$\frac{G_m}{G_m^0} = 2.71 + 0.242 \log [Ca]_i; \quad [Ca]_i \geq 10^{-7} M$$

(11)

where G_m^0 = the resting membrane conductance

Injection of calcium salts less than $10^{-7} M$ concentration causes no increase in G_m. Above this level, the conductance has a logarithmic dependency on $[Ca]_i$. Using the photoprotein aequorin as an intracellular calcium indicator, Eckert and Tillotson (1978) measured the effect of calcium entry during membrane depolarization on the late (potassium) currents. They concluded that activation of the late Ca^{2+}-dependent potassium current is causally related to the intracellular concentration of free calcium ions. This observation provides a functional interpretation of the Ca^{2+}-activated current: In neurons or muscle fibers with an inward calcium current during periods of activity and depolarization, the outward K^+ current opposes the action of the Ca^{2+} current and acts as a kind of negative feedback. This mechanism probably acts to stop the firing of action potentials in spontaneously active neurons with bursting discharge patterns (Chapter 9).

PROBLEMS

1. Using the following parameters of the Hodgkin-Huxley variable n, plot Cole and Moore's expression for the potassium conductance (Equation 1) for a period of 10 msec. What is the final value of g_K?

$$n_\infty = 0.983$$
$$n_0 = 0.315$$
$$\tau_n = 1.70 \text{ msec}$$
$$\bar{g}_K = 24.3 \text{ mS/cm}^2$$

2. Moore et al. (1967) showed that, to block the sodium channels in some lobster nerves, it takes about 1.6×10^{-11} moles of TTX per gram of nerve. How many molecules per gram of nerve are required to block?

3. Light and electron microscopic studies have shown that these lobster nerves have a total membrane area of about 0.7×10^4 cm^2/g. How many TTX molecules per square micrometer of nerve are required to block the sodium channels? (If at least one TTX molecule is required to block each sodium channel, this figure represents an upper limit to the number of Na^+ channels per square micrometer of membrane.)

4. In the node of Ranvier, Nonner et al. (1975) calculated a maximum gating charge transfer of 17,200 $e/\mu m^2$ during a depolarizing step. If six charges are assumed to cross the membrane for each gate that opens, what is the density of gates per square micrometer?

5. If the peak sodium conductance in the node in Problem 4 is 1.5 to 2.0 S/cm^2 (very high compared to squid axon!), what is the single-channel conductance?

6. In Connor and Stevens's expression for early outward current (Equation 10), some typical parameters during a step from a negative holding potential are

$$K = 200 \text{ nA}$$
$$\tau_A = 19 \text{ msec}$$
$$N = 4$$
$$\tau_B = 350 \text{ msec}$$

Plot I_A for the first 70 msec of the response.

REFERENCES

Armstrong, C. M. 1975. Ionic pores, gates, and gating currents. *Q. Rev. Biophys.* 7, 179–210.

Armstrong, C. M. and Bezanilla, F. 1973. Currents related to movement of the gating particles of the sodium channels. *Nature (Lond).* 242, 459–461.

Armstrong, C. M. and Bezanilla, F. 1974. Charge movement associated with the opening and closing of the activation gates of the Na channels. *J. Gen. Physiol.* 63, 533–552.

Armstrong, C. M., Bezanilla, F. and Rojas, E. 1973. Destruction of sodium conductance inactivation in squid axons perfused with pronase. *J. Gen. Physiol.* 62, 375–391.

Armstrong, C. M. and Binstock, L. 1965. Anomalous rectification in the squid giant axon injected with tetraethylammonium chloride. *J. Gen. Physiol.* 48, 859–872.

Bezanilla, F. and Armstrong, C. M. 1974. Gating currents of the sodium channels: three ways to block them. *Science* 183, 753–754.

Brodwick, M. S. and Junge, D. 1972. Post-stimulus hyperpolarization and slow potassium conductance increase in *Aplysia* giant neurone. *J. Physiol.* 223, 549–570.

Brown, A. M., Brodwick, M. S. and Eaton, D. C. 1977. Intracellular calcium and extraretinal photoreception in *Aplysia* giant neurons. *J. Neurobiol.* 8, 1–18.

Cole, K. S. and Moore, J. W. 1960. Potassium ion current in the squid giant axon: dynamic characteristic. *Biophys. J.* 1, 1–14.

Colquhoun, D., Henderson, R. and Ritchie, J. M. 1972. The binding of labeled tetrodotoxin to non-myelinated nerve fibres. *J. Physiol.* 227, 95–126.

Connor, J. A. and Stevens, C. F. 1971a. Voltage clamp studies of a transient outward membrane current in gastropod neural somata. *J. Physiol.* 213, 21–30.

Connor, J. A. and Stevens, C. F. 1971b. Prediction of repetitive firing behaviour from voltage clamp data on an isolated neurone soma. *J. Physiol.* 213, 31–53.

Eaton, D. C., Brodwick, M. S., Oxford, G. S. and Rudy, B. 1978. Arginine-specific reagents remove sodium channel inactivation. *Nature (Lond.)* 271, 473–476.

Eckert, R. and Tillotson, D. 1978. Potassium activation associated with intraneuronal free calcium. *Science* 200, 437–439.

Goldman, D. E. 1964. A molecular structural basis for the excitation properties of axons. *Biophys. J.* 4, 167–188.

Goldman, L. 1975. Pronase and models for the sodium conductance. *J. Gen. Physiol.* 65, 551–552.

Hafemann, D. R. 1972. Binding of radioactive tetrodotoxin to nerve membrane preparations. *Biochim. Biophys. Acta* 266, 548–556.

Hagiwara, S., Kusano, K. and Saito, N. 1961. Membrane changes of *Onchidium* nerve cell in potassium-rich media. *J. Physiol.* 155, 470–489.

Hagiwara, S. and Saito, N. 1959. Voltage-current relations in nerve cell membrane of *Onchidium verruculatum*. *J. Physiol.* 148, 161–179.

Hille, B. 1967. The selective inhibition of delayed potassium currents in nerve by tetraethylammonium ion. *J. Gen. Physiol.* 50, 1287–1302.

Hille, B. 1972. The permeability of the sodium channel to metal cations in myelinated nerve. *J. Gen. Physiol.* 59, 637–658.

Hille, B. 1978. Ionic channels in excitable membranes: current problems and biophysical approaches. *Biophys. J.* 22, 283–294.

Hille, B., Courtney, K. and Dum, R. 1975. Rate and site of action of local anesthetics in myelinated nerve fibers. *Molecular Mechanisms of Anesthesia*. B. R. Fink (ed.). New York, Raven, 13–20.

Hodgkin, A. L. and Huxley, A. F. 1952. A quantitative description of membrane current and its application to conduction and excitation in nerve. *J. Physiol.* 117, 500–544.

Hoyt, R. C. 1963. The squid giant axon: mathematical models. *Biophys. J.* 3, 399–431.

Keynes, R. D. and Rojas, E. 1974. Kinetics and steady-state properties of the charged system controlling sodium conductance in the squid giant axon. *J. Physiol.* 239, 393–434.

Levinson, S. R. and Meves, H. 1975. The binding of tritiated tetrodotoxin to squid giant axons. *Phil. Trans. R. Soc. B* 270, 349–352.

Meech, R. W. 1972. Intracellular calcium injection causes increased potassium conductance in *Aplysia* nerve cells. *Comp. Biochem. Physiol.* 42A, 493–499.

Meech, R. W. 1974. Calcium influx induces a post-tetanic hyperpolarization in *Aplysia* neurones. *Comp. Biochem. Physiol.* 48A, 387–395.

Meech, R. W. and Standen, N. B. 1975. Potassium activation in *Helix aspersa* neurones under voltage clamp: a component mediated by calcium influx. *J. Physiol.* 249, 211–239.

Meech, R. W. and Strumwasser, F. 1970. Intracellular calcium injection activates potassium conductance in *Aplysia* nerve cells. *Fed. Proc.* 29, 834.

Meves, H. 1974. The effect of holding potential on the asymmetry currents in squid giant axons. *J. Physiol.* 243, 847–867.

Moore, J. W., Anderson, N., Blaustein, M., Takata, M., Lettvin, J. Y., Pickard, W. F., Bernstein, T. and Pooler, J. 1966. Alkali cation selectivity of squid axon membrane. *Ann. N. Y. Acad. Sci.* 137, 818–829.

Moore, J. W., Narahashi, T. and Shaw, T. I. 1967. An upper limit to the number of sodium channels in nerve membrane? *J. Physiol.* 188, 99–105.

Mounier, Y. and Vassort, G. 1975. Evidence for a transient potassium membrane current dependent on calcium influx in crab muscle fiber. *J. Physiol.* 251, 609–625.

Mullins, L. J. 1959. An analysis of conductance changes in squid axon. *J. Gen. Physiol.* 42, 1013–1035.

Nakamura, Y., Nakajima, S. and Grundfest, H. 1965. The action of tetrodotoxin on electrogenic components of squid giant axons. *J. Gen. Physiol.* 48, 985–996.

Neher, E. 1971. Two fast transient current components during voltage clamp on snail neurons. *J. Gen. Physiol.* 58, 36–53.

Nonner, W., Rojas, E. and Stämpfli, R. 1975. Displacement currents in the node of Ranvier. *Pflügers Arch. Gesamte Physiol. Menschen Tiere* 354, 1–18.

Ritchie, J. M. and Rogart, R. B. 1977. Density of sodium channels in mammalian myelinated nerve fibers and the nature of the axonal membrane under the myelin sheath. *Proc. Natl. Acad. Sci. USA* 74, 211–215.

Rojas, E. and Rudy, B. 1976. Destruction of the sodium conductance inactivation by a specific protease in perfused nerve fibres from *Loligo*. *J. Physiol.* 262, 501–531.

Strichartz, G. R. 1973. The inhibition of sodium currents in myelinated nerve by quaternary derivatives of lidocaine. *J. Gen. Physiol.* 62, 37–57.

Taylor, R. E. 1959. Effect of procaine on electrical properties of squid axon membrane. *Am. J. Physiol.* 196, 1071–1078.

Tasaki, I. 1968. *Nerve Excitation: A Macromolecular Approach*. Springfield, Ill., Thomas.

Thompson, S. H. 1977. Three pharmacologically distinct potassium channels in molluscan neurones. *J. Physiol.* 265, 465–488.

8

CALCIUM CONDUCTANCES AND
ACTION POTENTIALS

DIVALENT SPIKES AND BI-IONIC POTENTIALS

The sodium hypothesis of nerve and muscle excitation was so important and convincing that for a number of years scientists continued to find only sodium-dependent action potentials in excitable membranes. However, in 1953 Fatt and Katz observed that action potentials could be seen in crab muscle fibers in Na^+-free solutions as long as calcium or magnesium ions were present in the external solution. They suggested that Ca^{2+} or Mg^{2+} might act as the inward current carrier.

In 1958, Fatt and Ginsborg performed some external ion substitutions with crayfish muscle fibers and concluded that neither sodium nor magnesium was essential for the production of action potentials; only external calcium was indispensable. These authors found that replacement of Ca^{2+} with Sr^{2+} or Ba^{2+} caused even larger action potentials than were seen with the normal amount of Ca^{2+}. Consequently, they developed a theory of divalent-ion action potentials that was based largely on strontium spikes. They assumed that when all the external calcium was replaced with strontium, the principal inward current through the membrane was due to Sr^{2+} and the principal outward current to K^+. By equating these currents at the peak of the action potential, they obtained the relationship

$$\frac{P_{Sr}[Sr]_o}{P_K[K]_i} = \frac{e^{EF/RT}(e^{EF/RT} + 1)}{4} \tag{1}$$

where P_{Sr} = strontium permeability
   P_K = potassium permeability
   $[Sr]_o$ = external strontium concentration
   $[K]_i$ = internal potassium concentration
   E = membrane potential at peak of spike
   R = universal gas constant
   T = temperature, K
   F = Faraday constant

While this equation cannot be solved explicitly for E, it permits plotting $[Sr]_o$ as a function of E. One feature of this equation is that the slope of the curve of E versus ln $[Sr]_o$ changes with E. (This is not true of a "pure-strontium" electrode, for which E is given by

$$E = \frac{RT}{2F} \ln \frac{[Sr]_o}{[Sr]_i} \qquad (2)$$

In this case the slope of E versus ln $[Sr]_o$ is constant.) In Equation 1, when E is large and negative,

$$\frac{P_{Sr}[Sr]_o}{P_K[K]_i} = \frac{e^{EF/RT}}{4} \qquad (3)$$

and

$$E = \frac{RT}{F} \ln \frac{4P_{Sr}[Sr]_o}{P_K[K]_i} \qquad (4)$$

This has a slope of 58 mV per tenfold change in $[Sr]_o$. When E is large and positive, Equation 1 becomes

$$\frac{P_{Sr}[Sr]_o}{P_K[K]_i} = \frac{e^{2EF/RT}}{4} \qquad (5)$$

and

$$E = \frac{RT}{2F} \ln \frac{4P_{Sr}[Sr]_o}{P_K[K]_i} \qquad (6)$$

This has a slope of 29 mV per tenfold change in $[Sr]_o$, like Equation 2. The variation of E with $[Sr]_o$ over a large range is shown in Figure 1.

This treatment was an application of the Nernst-Planck electro-diffusion model (Chapter 3) at a time when $dE/dt = 0$, so the membrane capacitive current was zero. It was referred to as the BI-IONIC

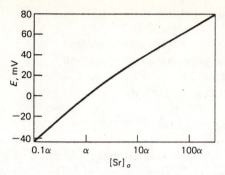

Graph of Equation 1, showing theoretical variation of action-potential over-shoot, E, with external strontium concentration, $[Sr]_o$. $\alpha = P_K[K]_i/2P_{Sr}$, defined in Equation 1. (From Fatt and Ginsborg, 1958.)

POTENTIAL THEORY, because the potential was determined by inward Sr^{2+} and outward K^+ currents occurring at the same time.

CALCIUM SPIKES

In 1964, Hagiwara, Naka, and others in California began to explore the ionic dependency of the action potential in the giant muscle fiber of the barnacle, *Balanus nubilis* Darwin. This exceedingly convenient preparation consisted of single muscle cells that often attained 4 cm in length and 2 mm in diameter. These huge fibers could easily be impaled with longitudinal electrodes, and the internal sarcoplasm could be replaced with buffered solutions having desired ion concentrations.

A few of the early observations that Hagiwara et al. made about the barnacle muscle fibers included that (1) usually no all-or-none action potential was produced by depolarizing these fibers in normal conditions, but (2) when the internal Ca^{2+} concentration was reduced by injecting some calcium chelating agent such as ethylene glycol bis (β-amino-ethylether)-N,N'-tetraacetic acid (EGTA), then all-or-none spikes could be reliably produced. Also, (3) replacement of external sodium with Tris (tris-hydroxymethyl aminomethane) had no effect on the all-or-none spike, and (4) the amplitude of the spike varied with external Ca^{2+} concentration and internal K^+ concentration in perfused fibers. This last behavior is illustrated in Figure 2. Columns A, B, and C were obtained from fibers injected with solutions of decreasing K^+ concentration, 485, 48, and 0 mM, respectively. Rows 1, 2, and 3 were obtained from these fibers in external solutions contain-

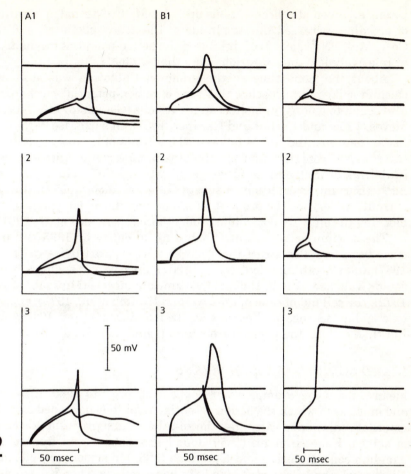

Variation of barnacle muscle action potential with external calcium concentration and internal potassium concentration. Subthreshold stimuli applied in several pictures. (From Hagiwara et al., 1964.)

ing, respectively, 20, 85, and 338 mM Ca^{2+}. The spikes were very much prolonged with K$^+$-free internal solutions, but in all cases the overshoot varied directly with log [Ca]$_o$ and inversely with log [K]$_i$. This result indicated that the membrane permeability to K$^+$ was substantial compared with that to Ca^{2+} during the peak of the spike.

Some other properties of calcium spikes that were unlike those of sodium spikes had been observed by Hagiwara and the earlier workers, including (1) that tetrodotoxin (TTX) had no effect on the action potentials, even at concentrations up to 1 mM, (2) external application of procaine increased the amplitude of the action potential, and (3) Co^{2+}, Mn^{2+}, Ni^{2+}, and La^{3+} inhibited the action-potential mechanism at relatively low concentrations (less than 20 mM).

About the same time as the group in California was studying calcium spikes in barnacles, this type of action-potential mechanism also began to emerge in molluscan nerve cells (Gerasimov et al., 1965; Meves, 1966; and Kerkut and Gardner, 1967). In each case with molluscan neurons, the spikes followed the criteria of (1) insensitivity to external Na^+ concentration or tetrodotoxin, (2) variation with external [Ca], [Ba], or [Sr], and (3) blockage by external Co^{2+}, Mn^{2+}, Ni^{2+}, or La^{3+}. (Barium, in addition to substituting for calcium as an inward current carrier, has the property of prolonging the action potential by blocking the outward potassium conductance [Sperelakis et al., 1967].)

The calcium spike was established as an entity by 1965 and has since been found in structures such as mussel heart (Irisawa et al., 1967) and smooth muscle (Twarog, 1967), presynaptic endings in the squid (Katz and Miledi, 1967, 1969), tunicate muscle (Miyazaki et al., 1972), the cell membrane of *Paramecium* (Naitoh et al., 1972), embryonic spinal neurons in *Xenopus* (Spitzer and Baccaglini, 1976), and Purkinje cells in the pigeon cerebellum (Llinás and Hess, 1976).

MIXED SODIUM-CALCIUM SPIKES

Meanwhile, some examples were appearing prior to 1965 of nerves and muscles in which the action potential amplitude depended on both external sodium and calcium—the so-called MIXED-DEPENDENCY class of spikes. Koketsu et al. (1959) found this behavior in frog spinal ganglion cells; Bülbring and Kuriyama (1963) in smooth muscle, and Niedergerke and Orkand (1966a,b) in heart muscle. Then Kerkut and Gardner (1967) and Junge (1967) described some molluscan neurons in which both sodium and calcium contributed to the action potential amplitude. This is illustrated in Figure 3, obtained with the R2 cell in *Aplysia*. The top row shows the action potential amplitude in normal saline (NS), sodium-free (Tris) solution, and normal saline afterward. The middle row shows the spike in normal saline, calcium-free (Tris) solution, and normal afterward. The bottom row shows normal, sodium- and calcium-free, and normal afterward. An all-or-none spike could be obtained in sodium-free or calcium-free solution for hours. However, replacement of both the external Na^+ and Ca^{2+} blocked the spike within 5 min, and the spike returned upon replacement of Na^+ or Ca^{2+} in the external solution. This mixed-dependency spike in *Aplysia* evidently arises from two different kinds of ionic channels;

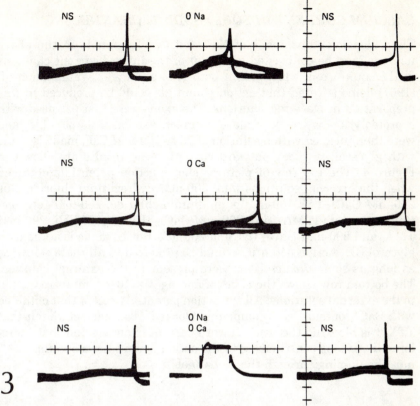

3 Variation of spike overshoot with external sodium and calcium concentration in *Aplysia* cell body. Sodium and calcium replaced with Tris. NS, normal saline; 0 Na, sodium-free; 0 Ca, calcium-free. Subthreshold stimuli applied in several pictures. (From Geduldig and Junge, 1968.)

this conclusion is based on three lines of evidence: (1) the Na^+ spike in Ca^{2+}-free solution is blocked by TTX but not by cobalt, (2) the Ca^{2+} spike in Na^+-free medium is blocked by cobalt but not by TTX (Geduldig and Junge, 1968), and (3) Geduldig and Gruener (1970) observed inward Ca^{2+} currents in voltage-clamped *Aplysia* neurons in Na^+-free solutions or in the presence of TTX. The Ca^{2+} currents were about one-tenth as large as the Na^+ currents and had a significantly slower time course. A similar separation of Na^+ and Ca^{2+} currents into different channels has been suggested for secretory cells in the crayfish eyestalk x-organ (Iwasaki and Satow, 1971) and in *Helix* A-cells (Standen, 1975a,b).

CALCIUM CURRENT IN SQUID SODIUM CHANNELS

The independent behavior of Na^+ and Ca^{2+} channels in the above neurons is to be contrasted with that of the inward-current channels in the squid axon, which admit both Na^+ and Ca^{2+}. Watanabe et al. (1967) demonstrated that action potentials could be produced in this preparation in Na^+-free solutions. The axons were first perfused with a proteolytic enzyme to remove as much axoplasm as possible, and were then injected with a solution of 25 to 100-mM CsF, made isotonic with glycerol, to block outward currents. The results are shown in Figure 4. The top row of pictures shows action potentials obtained when the external solutions were 300-mM hydrazinium chloride plus 200-mM $CaCl_2$ (A); 100-mM guanidinium chloride, 200-mM tetramethylammonium (TMA), and 200-mM $CaCl_2$ (B); 10-mM KCl, 290-mM TMA, and 200-mM $CaCl_2$ (C); and 200-mM $BaCl_2$, made isotonic with glycerol (D). Action potentials could be produced in all these solutions as long as some *divalent* ions were present in the external solution. The bottom row shows the effect of adding 2×10^{-8} g/ml tetrodotoxin to the external solutions. All the action potentials except that obtained with $BaCl_2$ outside were completely blocked. Watanabe et al. felt that TTX was blocking the usual inward-current channels and that therefore all the ions contributing to the action potentials, including Ca^{2+}, must be passing through those channels.

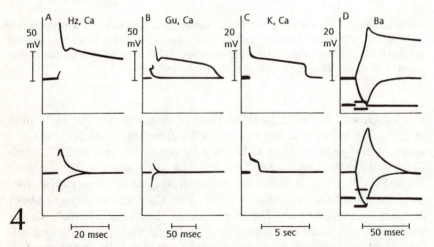

4

Spike activity in squid axon in sodium-free solutions. Top row: Various solutions as described in text. Bottom row: Effect of tetrodotoxin on action potentials in above solutions. (From Watanabe et al., 1967.)

This curious result was confirmed and explained convincingly in a voltage-clamp study reported by Meves and Vogel in 1973. These authors showed *two* components of inward Na^+ current in the squid axon: The first corresponded to Hodgkin and Huxley's inward current (up to a few milliamperes per square centimeter), and the second was much longer-lasting (time constant 14 msec at 17°C) and much smaller (tens of microamperes per square centimeter). In Na^+-free solutions containing 100-mM $CaCl_2$, Meves and Vogel observed inward Ca^{2+} currents with the same time course as the slow phase of the Na^+ current. The Ca^{2+} currents were blocked by TTX and were presumably going through the Na^+ channels. These slow divalent currents could explain the types of action potentials seen in the squid axon in Na^+-free solutions by Watanabe et al. (1967).

INTRACELLULAR CALCIUM INDICATORS

The first direct demonstration of calcium entry during the action potential in nerves and muscles was obtained with the calcium-sensitive protein aequorin. This substance, obtained from a luminescent jellyfish, was injected into excitable cells, where it emitted blue light in the presence of ionized calcium. Thus, by recording the emitted light with a photomultiplier tube, it was possible to follow dynamic changes in intracellular Ca^{2+} concentration (Ashley and Ridgway, 1970; Baker et al., 1971). The light signal does not vary linearly with calcium concentration but as a power function over a large range of concentrations (Tsien and Rink, 1983). One result obtained with the squid axon is shown in Figure 5. Curve A is the light resulting from a step depolarization of an axon injected with aequorin, as a function of the duration of the step; the longer the step, the greater the calcium entry. The rapid phase of Ca^{2+} entry is completed in about 200 msec. Curve B was obtained after application of TTX, which blocked the rapid phase but left intact a slower phase. Baker et al. (1971) showed that the rapid phase had about the same time course as the inward Na^+ current. This, together with the TTX result, indicated that the rapid phase was due to Ca^{2+} permeability of the sodium channels (about 1% of the Na^+ permeability). The slow phase was shown to resemble the known Ca^{2+} current in presynaptic terminals of the squid stellate synapse (Katz and Miledi, 1967, 1969). Both the synaptic current and the slow axonal current are insensitive to TTX and TEA, and both are blocked by Mg^{2+} or Mn^{2+} ions in the external solution.

Aequorin was then used to study intracellular calcium changes in presynaptic terminals in the squid synapse (Llinás et al., 1972), in *Aplysia* ganglion cell bodies (Stinnakre and Tauc, 1973), in *Limulus*

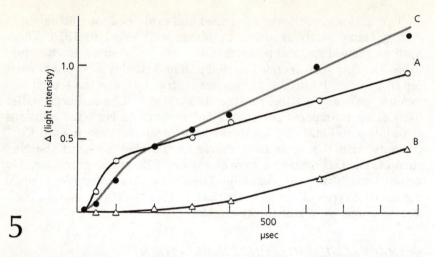

5

Two phases of calcium entry in squid axon. Aequorin injected into axon emits light with increasing internal Ca^{2+} concentration. Curve A: Light in response to voltage-clamp commands of increasing duration. Curve B: Same after application of 0.8-μM TTX. Curve C: After removal of TTX. Light intensity (Δ) is light normalized with respect to that produced by action potential, to compensate for changes with time. (From Baker et al., 1971.)

photoreceptors (Brown and Blinks, 1974), and in *Xenopus* muscle fibers (Taylor et al., 1975), among others. The main problem with this technique, apart from the difficulty of purifying the photoprotein and keeping it away from contaminating Ca^{2+} ions, was the relatively slow response time: The calcium-aequorin reaction has a half-time of a few msec (Hastings et al., 1969), which limits the ability to detect very rapid changes in Ca^{2+} concentration.

A faster method was then developed, using metallochromic dyes in which absorption of light changes very quickly upon exposure to calcium. With ARSENAZO III, for instance, the calcium-dye complexation takes less than 400 μsec (Brown et al., 1975). Changes in intracellular Ca^{2+} concentration may be monitored by injecting the arsenazo III into the structure of interest and measuring the amount of light transmitted under different conditions with a photodiode. This method has been successfully used with photoreceptors of *Limulus* to measure internal calcium changes during illumination (Brown et al., 1977). In the *Aplysia* R15 cell, it was used to follow changes in Ca^{2+} concentration during and between bursts of action potentials (Gorman and Thomas, 1978). These authors suggested that the internal calcium activated a strong membrane K conductance and that the interburst interval was determined by the time required to reduce the Ca^{2+} concentration (and K conductance) after each burst. Ahmed and Connor (1979) have used arsenazo III to monitor calcium concentration in voltage-clamped neurons of *Archidoris*. They found that increases in internal calcium during depolarizations resulted from influx and not from emptying of intracellular stores.

A probe with greater Ca^{2+}-sensitivity and higher selectivity for Ca^{2+} over Mg^{2+} was developed in 1985 by Grynkiewicz et al., a tetracarboxylate-based fluorescent indicator known as FURA-2. This compound is injected or soaked into neurons, muscle fibers, or other structures, then excited with light at wavelengths of 340 or 380 nm. The fluorescent signal (at 510 nm) with 340 nm excitation increases with increasing $[Ca]_i$. The emission with 380 nm light decreases with $[Ca]_i$. The ratio of the fluorescence with excitation at 340 and 380 nm increases linearly with calcium concentration. This technique has been used to demonstrate the presence of calcium channels in myelinated axons of the optic nerve (Lev-Ram and Grinvald, 1987), to show that inositol trisphosphate causes release of stored Ca^{2+} in *Aplysia* neurons (Fink et al., 1988), and to measure presynaptic increases in $[Ca]_i$ with posttetanic potentiation in crayfish motor nerve terminals (Delaney et al., 1989). Further applications of indicators such as these will undoubtedly add much more information about the functional role of intracellular calcium.

SIGNIFICANCE OF CALCIUM SPIKES

In nerve cells, calcium spikes may play a role in neurosecretion: Calcium-dependent action potentials have been found in sympathetic ganglion cells (Koketsu et al., 1959), in squid presynaptic endings (Katz and Miledi, 1967, 1969), and in crayfish neurosecretory cells (Iwasaki and Satow, 1971). Calcium ions are also necessary for the release of vasopressin in the pituitary (Douglas and Poisner, 1964).

In muscle cells from invertebrates, contraction often occurs without any regenerative action potentials. However, when action potentials do occur (with reduced intracellular Ca^{2+} concentration or following treatment with procaine or TEA), they are calcium spikes (Fatt and Katz, 1953; Fatt and Ginsborg, 1958; Hagiwara and Naka, 1964; and Hagiwara et al., 1964). Reversal of ciliary beating in paramecia has been shown to result from an increased Ca^{2+} conductance (Naitoh et al., 1972). Apparently, Ca^{2+} currents across excitable membranes occur in connection with EFFECTORS, i.e., secretory or contractile structures.

In vertebrate muscle fibers, the action potential is sodium dependent (Nastuk and Hodgkin, 1950) and apparently serves to conduct the impulse throughout the cell to provide uniform excitation. Sodium spikes in vertebrate nerves also conduct impulses over some distance. The calcium spikes seen in effectors may have the function of admitting calcium into the cells in order to activate some physiological mechanism.

REGULATION OF INTRACELLULAR CALCIUM CONCENTRATION

In experiments with indicators such as aequorin, arsenazo III, or fura-2, it is the concentration of free (ionized) calcium in the cytoplasm that is measured. This level results from the distribution of calcium among at least two intracellular compartments and the extracellular compartment, as shown in Figure 6. The heavy arrow indicates calcium entry, either passive or as a result of activity. This calcium may be extruded via an active "calcium pump" or in exchange for sodium; it may be taken up by mitochondria or it may bind with other intracellular systems such as sarcoplasmic reticulum in muscle or inorganic

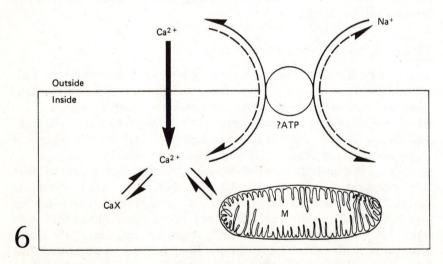

Distribution of calcium ion between outside and inside of nerve cell. Ionized Ca^{2+} concentration determined by rate of influx (heavy arrow), extrusion by Na^+/Ca^{2+} exchange and calcium pump, uptake by mitochondria (M), and binding to intracellular binding systems (X). (From Baker and Glitsch, 1975.)

anions. The amount measured by an indicator is that left in the cytoplasm after the rest has been distributed.

Hodgkin and Keynes (1957) used $^{45}Ca^{2+}$ to trace the efflux and influx during activity of the squid axon. The efflux was estimated by comparing loss of activity in stimulated and unstimulated axons that had been injected with isotope. It apparently did not change with activity. The influx was compared in stimulated and unstimulated axons by counting the activity of extruded axoplasm. By this means, Hodgkin and Keynes found an extra uptake of Ca^{2+} per impulse of 0.006 pmol/cm^2. (This compares with a sodium uptake of about 4 pmol/cm^2 or about 667 times that of calcium.) The entry of calcium per impulse varied approximately linearly with external Ca^{2+} concentration. The resting influx in the squid axon has more recently been estimated at about 0.1–0.2 pmol/cm^2/sec (Brinley et al., 1975), so the extra influx produced by 100 spikes in one sec (0.6 pmol/cm^2) is significantly larger than the basal level.

The resting intracellular concentration of calcium has been found to be quite low compared to that of other ions inside or outside of cells. Hagiwara and Nakajima (1966) estimated a value of 100 nM for the barnacle giant muscle fiber by noting the effects of injected buffers with known Ca^{2+} concentration on excitation-contraction coupling. Meech (1974) found a value close to 500 nM for *Helix* neurons while examining the effect of injected buffers on the calcium-activated potassium conductance. Baker (1972) suggested a value close to 100 nM for squid axon, although Dipolo et al. (1976) lowered this to 20–50 nM. Further references to intracellular calcium concentrations in the range 1–700 nM measured with Ca^{2+}-sensitive electrodes may be found in the reference by Tsien and Rink (1983).

Given the known influx of calcium, these low levels inside neurons and muscles require that an outward flux must also be present. Since the external concentration is normally in the range 1–11 mM, the concentration gradient for calcium is of the order of 10^5 and the electrical gradient tends to drive calcium into the cell. Thus, calcium must be extruded by some sort of active process.

The presence of an ATP-dependent calcium pump in nerve was in question for several years. Blaustein and Hodgkin (1969) observed an increase in Ca^{2+} efflux when cyanide, which blocks ATP production, was applied to the squid axon. This contradicted the idea of an ATP-driven outward pump, and the effect was later attributed to the unloading of Ca^{2+} from intracellular binding sites (probably mitochondria). An alternate explanation of Ca^{2+} extrusion was found by Baker et al. (1967). The influx of $^{45}Ca^{2+}$ into squid axons increased and the efflux decreased if the transmembrane sodium gradient was decreased.

Blaustein and Hodgkin (1969) also found that the Ca^{2+} efflux increased with increasing sodium gradient. This suggested that extrusion of calcium was coupled with entry of sodium in an EXCHANGE DIFFUSION (counter-transport) process. The energy for calcium to move "uphill" against a gradient was provided by the "downhill" movement of sodium. A similar behavior was found in heart muscle by Reuter and Seitz (1968). Blaustein and Russell (1975) also demonstrated a dependence of calcium efflux on external Na^+ and Ca^{2+} concentrations and calculated that for the Na^+/Ca^{2+} exchange one Ca^{2+} ion exchanges with three Na^+ ions. Finally, an ATP-dependent calcium extrusion has been shown in axons in which the Na^+/Ca^{2+} exchange is blocked with sodium-free external solution (Dipolo and Beaugé, 1979). Thus, three mechanisms may contribute to calcium efflux in squid axons: an ATP-dependent pump, Na^+/Ca^{2+} exchange, and Ca^{2+}/Ca^{2+} exchange. In muscle, the picture is slightly more complicated, since the additional intracellular calcium-binding compartment of the contractile apparatus must be included.

DEVELOPMENTAL CHANGES IN CALCIUM, SODIUM, AND POTASSIUM CHANNELS

An intriguing tool became available in the 1970s for dissecting out different ion channels in membranes: Apparently, the relative numbers of sodium-, calcium-, and potassium-selective channels changed during ontogenetic development in some animals. One example is shown in Figure 7, taken from tunicate muscle in different states (Takahashi et al., 1971). At the top, the all-or-none action potential in a tadpole with a 90% grown tail is shown; it has a duration of over 2 sec. At the bottom, obtained in a fully grown tadpole, the duration has shrunk to less than 0.1 sec. Evidently, the repolarization (K^+) channels have appeared at a later time than the depolarization channels. In a subsequent study Miyazaki et al. (1972) showed that the inward-current mechanism itself changes with time: Egg cells that are precursors of the tunicate muscles have action potentials that are dependent on both sodium and calcium ions. By the time the muscle cells are fully differentiated, the sodium current is suppressed and the spikes are dependent on Ca^{2+} only.

These studies indicated the potential for developmental changes in excitable membranes, and such changes were soon seen in other preparations. In a clonal culture of rat skeletal muscle, Kidokoro (1975) found an Na^+ component in myoblast action potentials, both Na^+ and Ca^{2+} components in the myotube stage, and only an Na^+ component

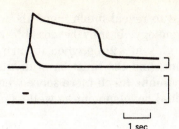

1 sec

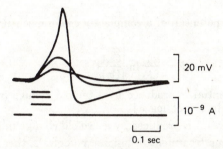

20 mV

10^{-9} A

0.1 sec

7

Differential development of spike plateau and repolarization mechanisms in tunicate muscle. Upper traces in each part show membrane potential, lower traces applied current. Top: Response of muscle cell of tadpole with 90% grown tail. Bottom: Response of muscle cell of fully grown tadpole after hatching. Same voltage and current calibrations in all parts. (From Takahashi et al., 1971.)

in the fully differentiated stage (like adult skeletal muscle in vivo). The Ca^{2+} component appeared for a while in these cells and then departed. Another pattern of development was seen in spinal cord neurons of *Xenopus* (Spitzer and Baccaglini, 1976; Baccaglini and Spitzer, 1977). At the earliest stages in which action potentials can be evoked, the inward current is carried by calcium only. Then a sodium current appears, and at intermediate stages the inward current is carried both by sodium and calcium. Finally the calcium current is eliminated and the inward current in adult neurons is carried by sodium only. In these cells, calcium spikes become sodium spikes.

These developmental changes in the mechanism of excitability may somewhat parallel the course of evolution; calcium action potentials are seen mainly in invertebrate neurons or muscle fibers and sodium spikes are seen more uniformly in the vertebrates. (Of course, there are exceptions, such as the squid axon and vertebrate spinal ganglion cell.) This approach promises to reveal much more about both development and membrane physiology: It may be possible to study one type of channel more thoroughly at a time when its currents are not masked by those of other ions, and the function of divalent currents in excitable membranes may make much more sense when viewed in an overall context of individual development as well as phylogeny.

PROBLEMS

1. The transmembrane potential of a completely calcium-sensitive electrode is given by

$$E = \frac{RT}{2F} \ln \frac{[Ca]_o}{[Ca]_i}$$

   What change in potential is produced by a tenfold change in $[Ca]_o$? [Remember that $(RT/F) \ln x = 58 \log x$.]

2. What change in potential is produced by a twofold change in $[Ca]_o$?

3. In Fatt and Ginsborg's treatment of bi-ionic potentials, there was no potassium in the external solution and negligible internal strontium. The currents for these two ions were then given by

$$I_{Sr} = 4P_{Sr} \frac{EF^2}{RT} \frac{[Sr]_o}{1 - e^{2EF/RT}}$$

$$I_K = -P_K \frac{EF^2}{RT} \frac{[K]_i e^{EF/RT}}{1 - e^{EF/RT}}$$

   They assumed that, at the peak of the action potential, $I_{Sr} + I_K = 0$. Show that this leads to Equation 1.

4. In Equation 1, how negative must E be in order that Equation 3 is a reasonable approximation? (You might take as a criterion that $e^{EF/RT} + 1 = 1.05$, i.e., approximately $= 1$.)

5. In the data of Figure 2, when $[K]_i = 48$ mM, the spike overshoot (OS) varied with $[Ca]_o$ as follows:

$[Ca]_o$, mM	OS, mV
20	6.9
85	27.5
338	47.5

   What is the approximate change in overshoot for a tenfold change in $[Ca]_o$?

6. The active region of a squid axon used in a calcium uptake study is 0.8 mm in diameter and 4 cm long. Using Hodgkin and Keynes's data for Ca^{2+} entry, calculate the expected increase per impulse in intracellular Ca^{2+} concentration in nM, assuming the calcium diffuses uniformly throughout the axon.

REFERENCES

Ahmed, Z. and Connor, J. A. 1979. Measurement of calcium influx under voltage clamp in molluscan neurones using the metallochromic dye arsenazo III. *J. Physiol.* 286, 61–82.

Ashley, C. C. and Ridgway, E. B. 1970. On the relationship between membrane potential, calcium transient and tension in single barnacle muscle fibres. *J. Physiol.* 209, 105–130.

Baccaglini, P. I. and Spitzer, N. C. 1977. Developmental changes in the inward current of the action potential of Rohon-Beard neurones. *J. Physiol.* 271, 93–117.

Baker, P. F. 1972. Transport and metabolism of calcium ions in nerve. *Prog. Biophys. Mol. Biol.* 24, 177–223.

Baker, P. F. and Glitsch, H. G. 1975. Voltage-dependent changes in the permeability of nerve membranes to calcium and other divalent cations. *Phil. Trans. R. Soc. B.* 270, 389–409.

Baker, P. F., Blaustein, M. P., Hodgkin, A. L. and Steinhardt, R. A. 1967. The effect of sodium concentration on calcium movements in giant axons of *Loligo forbesi. J. Physiol.* 192, 43–44P.

Baker, P. F., Hodgkin, A. L. and Ridgway, E. B. 1971. Depolarization and calcium entry in squid giant axons. *J. Physiol.* 218, 709–755.

Blaustein, M. P. and Hodgkin, A. L. 1969. The effect of cyanide on the efflux of calcium from squid axons. *J. Physiol.* 200, 497–527.

Blaustein, M. P. and Russell, J. M. 1975. Sodium-calcium exchange and calcium-calcium exchange in internally dialyzed squid giant axons. *J. Membr. Biol.* 22, 285–312.

Brinley, F. J., Spangler, S. G. and Mullins, L. J. 1975. Calcium and EDTA fluxes in dialyzed squid axons. *J. Gen. Physiol.* 66, 223–250.

Brown, J. E. and Blinks, J. R. 1974. Changes in intracellular free calcium during illumination of invertebrate photoreceptors: detection with aequorin. *J. Gen. Physiol.* 64, 643–665.

Brown, J. E., Cohen, L. B., De Weer, P., Pinto, L. H., Ross, W. N. and Salzberg, B. M. 1975. Rapid changes of intracellular free calcium concentration. *Biophys. J.* 15, 1155–1160.

Brown, J. E., Brown, P. K. and Pinto, L. H. 1977. Detection of light-induced changes of intracellular ionized calcium concentration in *Limulus* ventral photoreceptors using arsenazo III. *J. Physiol.* 267, 299–320.

Bülbring, E. and Kuriyama, H. 1963. Effects of changes in the external sodium and calcium concentrations on spontaneous electrical activity in smooth muscle of guinea pig *taenia coli. J. Physiol.* 166, 29–58.

Delaney, K. R., Zucker, R. S. and Tank, D. W. 1989. Calcium in motor nerve terminals associated with posttetanic potentiation. *J. Neuroscience* 9, 3558–3567.

Dipolo, R. and Beaugé, L. 1979. Physiological role of ATP-driven calcium pump in squid axon. *Nature (Lond.)* 278, 271–273.

Dipolo, R., Requena, J., Brinley, F. J., Mullins, L. J., Scarpa, A. and Tiffert, T. 1976. Ionized calcium concentrations in squid axons. *J. Gen. Physiol.* 67, 433–467.

Douglas, W. W. and Poisner, A. M. 1964. Stimulus-secretion coupling in a neurosecretory organ: the role of calcium in the release of vasopressin from the neurohypophysis. *J. Physiol.* 172, 1–18.

Fatt, P. and Ginsborg, B. L. 1958. The ionic requirements for the production of action potentials in crustacean muscle fibres. *J. Physiol.* 142, 516–543.

Fatt, P. and Katz, B. 1953. The electrical properties of crustacean muscle fibres. *J. Physiol.* 120, 171–204.

Fink, L. A., Connor, J. A. and Kaczmarek, L. K. 1988. Inositol trisphosphate releases intracellularly stored calcium and modulates ion channels in molluscan neurons. *J. Neuroscience.* 8, 2544–2555.

Geduldig, D. and Gruener, R. 1970. Voltage clamp of the *Aplysia* giant neurone: early sodium and calcium currents. *J. Physiol.* 211, 217–244.

Geduldig, D. and Junge, D. 1968. Sodium and calcium components of action potentials in the *Aplysia* giant neurone. *J. Physiol.* 199, 347–365.

Gerasimov, V. D., Kostyuk, P. G. and Maiskii, V. A. 1965. The influence of divalent cations on the electrical characteristics of membranes of giant neurones. *Biofizika* 10, 447–453.

Gorman, A. L. F. and Thomas, M. V. 1978. Changes in the intracellular concentration of free calcium ions in a pace-maker neurone, measured with the metallochromic indicator dye arsenazo III. *J. Physiol.* 275, 357–376.

Grynkiewicz, G., Poenie, M. and Tsien, R. Y. 1985. A new generation of Ca^{2+} indicators with greatly improved fluorescence properties. *J. Biol. Chem.* 260, 3440–3450.

Hagiwara, S. and Naka, K. 1964. The initiation of spike potential in barnacle muscle fibers under low intracellular Ca^{++}. *J. Gen. Physiol.* 48, 141–162.

Hagiwara, S. and Nakajima, S. 1966. Differences in Na and Ca spikes as examined by application of tetrodotoxin, procaine and manganese ions. *J. Gen. Physiol.* 49, 793–806.

Hagiwara, S., Chichibu, S. and Naka, K. 1964. The effects of various ions on resting and spike potentials of barnacle muscle fibers. *J. Gen. Physiol.* 48, 163–179.

Hastings, J. W., Mitchell, G., Mattingly, P. H., Blinks, J. R. and Van Leeuven, M. 1969. Response of aequorin bioluminescence to rapid changes in calcium concentration. *Nature (Lond.)* 222, 1047–1050.

Hodgkin, A. L. and Keynes, R. D. 1957. Movements of labelled calcium in squid giant axons. *J. Physiol.* 138, 253–281.

Irisawa, H., Shigeto, N. and Otani, M. 1967. Effect of Na^+ and Ca^{2+} on the excitation of the *Mytilus* (bivalve) heart muscle. *Comp. Biochem. Physiol.* 23, 199–212.

Iwasaki, S. and Satow, Y. 1971. Sodium- and calcium-dependent spike potentials in the secretory neuron soma of the x-organ of the crayfish. *J. Gen. Physiol.* 57, 216–238.

Junge, D. 1967. Multi-ionic action potentials in molluscan giant neurones. *Nature (Lond.)* 215, 546–548.

Katz, B. and Miledi, R. 1967. A study of synaptic transmission in the absence of nerve impulses. *J. Physiol.* 192, 407–436.

Katz, B. and Miledi, R. 1969. Tetrodotoxin-resistant electric activity in presynaptic terminals. *J. Physiol.* 203, 459–487.

Kerkut, G. A. and Gardner, D. R. 1967. The role of calcium ions in the action potentials of *Helix aspersa* neurones. *Comp. Biochem. Physiol.* 20, 147–162.

Kidokoro, Y. 1975. Sodium and calcium components of the action potential in a developing skeletal muscle cell line. *J. Physiol.* 244, 145–159.

Koketsu, K., Cerf, J. A. and Nishi, S. 1959. Further observations on the activity of frog spinal ganglion cells in sodium-free solutions. *J. Neurophysiol.* 22, 693–703.

Lev-Ram, V. and Grinvald, A. 1987. Activity-dependent calcium transients in central nervous system myelinated axons revealed by the calcium indicator FURA-2. *Biophys. J.* 52, 571–576.

Llinás, R. and Hess, R. 1976. Tetrodotoxin-resistant dendritic spikes in avian Purkinje cells. *Proc. Natl. Acad. Sci. USA* 73, 2520–2523.

Llinás, R., Blinks, J. R. and Nicholson, C. 1972. Calcium transients in presynaptic terminal of squid giant synapse: detection with aequorin. *Science* 176, 1127–1129.

Meech, R. W. 1974. The sensitivity of *Helix aspersa* neurones to injected calcium ions. *J. Physiol.* 237, 259–277.

Meves, H. 1966. Das Aktionspotential der Riesennervenzellen der Weinbergschnecke *Helix pomatia*. *Pflügers Arch. Gesamte Physiol. Menschen Tiere* 289, R10.

Meves, H. and Vogel, W. 1973. Calcium inward currents in internally perfused giant axons. *J. Physiol.* 235, 225–265.

Miyazaki, S., Takahashi, K. and Tsuda, K. 1972. Calcium and sodium contributions to regenerative response in the embryonic excitable cell membrane. *Science* 176, 1441–1443.

Naitoh, Y., Eckert, R. and Friedman, K. 1972. A regenerative calcium response in *Paramecium*. *J. Exp. Biol.* 56, 667–681.

Nastuk, W. L. and Hodgkin, A. L. 1950. The electrical activity of single muscle fibers. *J. Cell. Comp. Physiol.* 35, 39–73.

Niedergerke, R. and Orkand, R. K. 1966a. The dual effect of calcium on the action potential of the frog's heart. *J. Physiol.* 184, 291–311.

Niedergerke, R. and Orkand, R. K. 1966b. The dependence of the action potential of the frog's heart on the external and intracellular sodium concentration. *J. Physiol.* 184, 312–334.

Reuter, H. and Seitz, N. 1968. The dependence of calcium efflux from cardiac muscle on temperature and external ion composition. *J. Physiol.* 195, 451–470.

Sperelakis, N., Schneider, M. F. and Harris, E. J. 1967. Decreased K^+ conductance produced by Ba^{++} in frog sartorius fibers. *J. Gen. Physiol.* 50, 1565–1583.

Spitzer, N. C. and Baccaglini, P. I. 1976. Development of the action potential in embryo amphibian neurons *in vivo*. *Brain Res.* 107, 610–616.

Standen, N. B. 1975a. Calcium and sodium ions as charge carriers in the action potential of an identified snail neurone. *J. Physiol.* 249, 241–252.

Standen, N. B. 1975b. Voltage-clamp studies of the calcium inward current in an identified snail neurone: comparison with the sodium inward current. *J. Physiol.* 249, 253–268.

Stinnakre, J. and Tauc, L. 1973. Calcium influx in active *Aplysia* neurones detected by injected aequorin. *Nature New Biol.* 242, 113–115.

Takahashi, K., Miyazaki, S. and Kidokoro, Y. 1971. Development of excitability in embryonic muscle cell membranes in certain tunicates. *Science* 171, 415–418.

Taylor, S. R., Rüdel, R. and Blinks, J. R. 1975. Calcium transients in amphibian muscle. *Fed. Proc.* 34, 1379.

Tsien, R. Y. and Rink, T. J. 1983. Measurement of free Ca^{2+} in cytoplasm. *Current Methods in Cellular Neurobiology V. III: Electrophysiological and Optical Recording Techniques.* Barker, J. L., and McKelvy, J. F. (eds.). New York, Wiley, 249–312.

Twarog, B. M. 1967. Excitation of *Mytilus* smooth muscle. *J. Physiol.* 192, 857–868.

Watanabe, A., Tasaki, I., Singer, I. and Lerman, L. 1967. Effects of tetrodotoxin on excitability of squid giant axons in sodium-free media. *Science* 155, 95–97.

9

REPETITIVE FIRING

EXAMPLES OF RHYTHMICITY

Repetitive firing in excitable membranes has been of interest to physiologists at least since the 1920s (Adrian, 1928; Adrian and Gelfan, 1933; Fessard, 1936; Arvanitaki, 1939). It is associated with movement, secretion, the heartbeat, respiration, peristalsis, sensory perception, and circadian rhythms, among other things. It may occur spontaneously or in response to an applied stimulus (such as a maintained current, light, or mechanical displacement). An assortment of types of repetitive activity is shown in Figure 1, ranging in frequency from about 0.8 to 80 per sec. A and B are from "pacemaker" neurons in *Aplysia*, C is from a crab axon, D is from a lobster stretch receptor, and E is from cat intestinal muscle. In each case, a slow PACEMAKER POTENTIAL precedes and initiates the spike. This behavior is like that of a relaxation oscillator and can be modeled with a generalized oscillator theory (FitzHugh, 1961). Repetitive firing is a higher-order phenomenon than the production of action potentials in that knowledge of the roles of sodium and potassium in the spike mechanism is not sufficient to predict repetition. It is necessary to formulate a specific model with measured parameters (e.g., the Hodgkin-Huxley model or a modification of it) and see whether or not it predicts this behavior. The subject is thus a kind of justification for model-making, and in this chapter several different models will be examined.

148

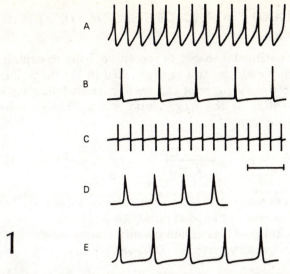

Repetitive activity in excitable cells. A and B: Pacemaker neurons in *Aplysia*. (From Junge and Moore, 1966.) C: Crab axon. (From Hodgkin, 1948.) D: Lobster stretch receptor. (From Calvin, 1978.) E: Cat intestinal muscle. (From Prosser, 1978.) Time scale: 0.67 sec in A and B; 0.24 sec in C: 15 msec in D; and 1.33 sec in E.

EFFECTS OF LOW-CALCIUM SOLUTIONS

It has been known for more than half a century that normally silent excitable cells can become spontaneously active if the external calcium concentration is lowered. This has been well documented in single muscle fibers (Adrian and Gelfan, 1933) and in axons of cuttlefish (Arvanitaki, 1939) and squid (Brink et al., 1946). Nowadays, we may understand this as resulting from either of two effects: (1) The conductance-voltage curve for the inward current may be shifted toward more negative potentials (Chapter 5). The electric field in the membrane becomes less than the critical gradient for excitation, and spontaneous activity is produced. This is probably a result of decreased screening of negative surface charges in low-calcium solutions (McLaughlin et al., 1971; D'Arrigo, 1973; Brismar, 1973; Begenisich, 1975). (2) The repetitive firing could also be due to a lowering of potassium conductance, secondary to a decrease in internal calcium concentration (Chapter 7). Either of these effects could explain the hyperexcitability and muscle twitching seen in patients with hypoparathyroidism, which lowers the blood calcium level.

REFRACTORINESS AND TWO-FACTOR THEORIES OF FIRING FREQUENCY

In 1928, E.D. Adrian outlined a theory of repetitive firing to explain the excitation of sensory endings; this is illustrated in Figure 2. The solid line shows the recovery curve of threshold current following a compound action potential in the frog sciatic nerve. This may be represented by the expression

$$I = I_{th} + \frac{0.0015}{T - T_r} \tag{1}$$

where I = stimulus current required to excite at any duration
I_{th} = threshold current at longest durations = 1
T = interval after previous action potential, sec
T_r = absolute refractory period = 0.002 sec

According to this theory, if a stimulus of strength $b_1, b_2, \ldots, b_n$ is applied, the nerve will be able to produce a second action potential

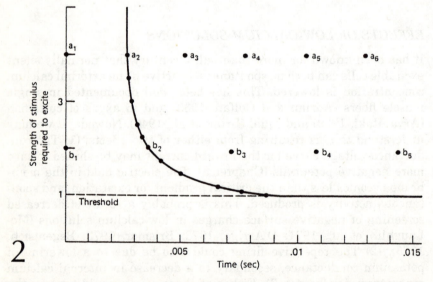

Refractoriness model of repetitive firing. Solid line shows threshold versus time after previous spike. Small stimulus b excites at longer interval than large stimulus a. (From Adrian, 1928.)

after about 0.0035 sec and will continue to fire repetitively at this interval. A stronger stimulus $a_1, a_2, \ldots, a_n$ will excite after only 0.0025 sec, and the repetition rate will be correspondingly faster. The interval between action potentials in the model is thus

$$T = 0.002 + \frac{0.0015}{I - 1} \tag{2}$$

where T and I are the same as in Equation 1.

The firing rates predicted by this theory were much higher than those actually observed in repetitively firing axons or sensory endings. Accordingly, some "two-factor" theories were produced in which both threshold and membrane potential or some other excitatory factor were assumed to vary following a spike (Rashevsky, 1933; Hill, 1936). A simple two-factor approach to repetitive firing is shown in Figure 3. V_m and V_t are the membrane potential and threshold, measured from the undershoot. They are given by

$$V_m = IR_m(1 - e^{-t/\tau_m}) \tag{3}$$

$$V_t = A/t + B \tag{4}$$

where I = applied current
      R_m = membrane resistance
      τ_m = membrane time constant
      A and B are constants

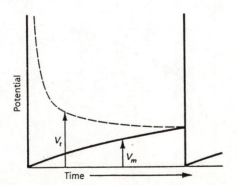

3

A two-factor model of repetitive firing. Solid line shows potential and broken line shows threshold versus time after previous spike. Next spike occurs when $V_m = V_t$.

A second spike is assumed to occur when $V_m = V_t$. Equations 3 and 4 may be solved simultaneously to find t, the interspike interval. By making V_t a rapid process as shown, the response time of the potential curve can be more important than refractoriness in determining the interval.

Various refinements were added to the two-factor models, e.g., a local response, or slow depolarization (which itself has a threshold [Hodgkin, 1948]), and accommodation to maintained stimuli (Fuortes and Mantegazzini, 1962). However, this type of analysis could never predict repetitive waveforms very accurately, perhaps because it did not take into account the close relationship between the mechanisms of the pacemaker and spike potentials. In order to do this, an overall model of the repetitive cell had to be constructed.

REPETITIVE DISCHARGE IN A MODEL AXON

Since the Hodgkin-Huxley theory was the first detailed description of current flows during excitation, it was the first such model to be applied to repetitive firing. Unfortunately, as shown by Stein (1967), it only predicts repetitive firing over a limited range of frequencies: Figure 4 shows the frequency-current relation for a spaced-clamped model axon at 6.3°C. Below a frequency of 50 action potentials (ap) per sec, the discharge falls off abruptly; and above 125 ap per sec, it degenerates into fast oscillations. The range of possible frequencies in the model becomes even smaller at higher temperatures: at 20°C, it

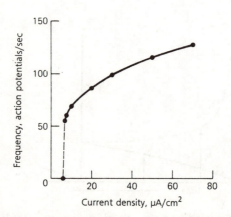

4

Current-frequency curve for repetitive firing in Hodgkin-Huxley model of uniformly polarized axon at 6.3°C. (From Stein, 1967.)

is about 200–280 ap per sec. These results corroborated the findings of Hagiwara and Oomura (1958) in real squid axons: At 14–18°C, repetitive discharge occurs only in the range 230–330 ap per sec. Clearly, neither the squid axon nor the original Hodgkin-Huxley theory is a good model for the very slow firing (less than 1 ap per sec) seen in some excitable cells.

In order to extend the range of firing frequencies, Shapiro and Lenherr (1972) and Kernell and Sjöholm (1973) added hypothetical potassium conductances, which did permit slower firing. Dodge (1972) shifted the potassium conductance parameters 8 mV in the positive direction; this reduced the potassium conductance and increased the subthreshold membrane resistance and time constant. This model allowed repetitive firing down to 10 ap per sec, but the frequency in the low range was extremely sensitive to stimulus strength.

MODELING THE MOLLUSCAN NEURON

One class of excitable cells that could fire repetitively at frequencies as low as 1 ap per second were the large nerve cell bodies found in mollusc ganglia. The action potentials in these structures differed from those in squid and crustacean axons in that they were longer in duration and often had large calcium components (Carpenter and Gunn, 1970; Chapter 8).

Alving (1969) found a curious difference between pacemaker and nonpacemaker neurons in *Aplysia* when long depolarizing steps were applied with a voltage clamp: The outward current in pacemakers reached an initial peak in 100 msec and then fell with a time constant of seconds, whereas that in nonpacemakers increased to a steady plateau. This difference was explained by Eaton (1972), who showed that during the voltage clamp step pacemaker cells undergo a positive shift in the potassium equilibrium potential due to K^+ accumulation outside the cells. This accumulation of potassium has been measured directly with ion-sensitive electrodes by Neher and Lux (1973). One difference between pacemakers and nonpacemakers may be that pacemakers have more extensively infolded membranes and retain more of the accumulated potassium in the infoldings.

Some quantitative understanding that pacemaker activity must include a periodic change in potassium *conductance* was available for many years in the field of cardiac physiology (Dudel and Trautwein, 1958; Trautwein and Kassebaum, 1961). This was suspected to be the case for *Aplysia* pacemakers as well (Alving, 1969; Carpenter and Gunn, 1970; Neher and Lux, 1971). The first model to incorporate periodic changes in membrane conductances to describe the activity of a molluscan cell body was that of Connor and Stevens (1971b). They used a modified Hodgkin-Huxley theory for the membrane current $I(t)$:

$$I(t) = C_m\frac{dE}{dt} + g_I(E - E_I) + g_K(E - E_K) + g_A(E - E_A) + g_l(E - E_l) \quad (5)$$

where C_m = membrane capacitance
$\quad\quad g_I$ = inward-current conductance (sodium and/or calcium)
$\quad\quad g_K$ = delayed potassium conductance
$\quad\quad g_A$ = early outward potassium conductance (as in Chapter 7)
$\quad\quad g_l$ = leak conductance
$\quad E_I, E_K, E_A$, and E_l are equilibrium potentials

To describe g_I, the inward-current conductance, they used

$$g_I(E,t) = \bar{g}_I A_I^3(E,t) B_I(E,t) \quad (6)$$

where $A_I(E,t)$ is analogous to the Hodgkin-Huxley m
$\quad\quad B_I(E,t)$ is analogous to h

Instead of giving systematic equations for A_I and B_I (as Hodgkin and Huxley did for m and h), Connor and Stevens used piecewise linear approximations to the measured curves of activation and inactivation parameters; thus the model parameters were the same as those observed. The other conductances were given by

$$g_K(E,t) = \bar{g}_K A_K^2(E,t) B_K(E,t) \quad (7)$$

$$g_A(E,t) = \bar{g}_A A_A^4(E,t) B_A(E,t) \quad (8)$$

$$g_l(E,t) = \text{constant} \quad (9)$$

The delayed potassium conductance $g_K(E,t)$ shows some inactivation (i.e., falling off at late times). The early outward conductance $g_A(E,t)$ has the form observed in these cells by Connor and Stevens (1971a). This current is activated at a lower threshold potential than the inward sodium current and requires a preceding hyperpolarization before the activating potential change. In Figure 5, Part A, the computed potential curve (asterisk) is compared to that seen in an *Anisodoris* cell. In Part B, the model currents that flow in the interspike interval are shown; the currents during the action potential are omitted. It can be seen that the early current I_A is dominant in the first part of the interval. This has the effect of slowing the rate of depolarization

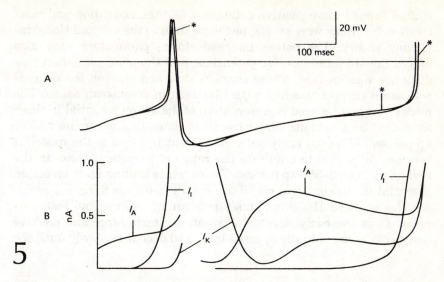

5

Potentials and ionic currents during repetitive firing in model of *Anisodoris* neuron. A: Computed (*) and observed pacemaker and action potentials. B: I_A, early outward current; I_I, inward current; I_K, delayed potassium current. Currents during action potential not shown. (From Connor and Stevens, 1971b.)

and allowing slow firing rates. As seen in Part A of this figure, the Connor-Stevens model gives a close representation of both the action potential and the interspike potential waveform in these pacemaker cells. It was the first detailed model based on measured cell parameters to do so.

OTHER AXONS

Another system that fires repetitively at low rates and in which the membrane ionic conductances can be measured under voltage-clamp conditions is the walking-leg axon of the crustaceans *Callinectes* and *Cancer*. This system has been studied by Connor and co-workers (Connor, 1975; Connor et al., 1977). These axons generate an early outward current like that found in molluscan nerve cell bodies (Connor and Stevens, 1971a; Neher, 1971; see Chapter 7).

In order to model the slow repetitive firing that is seen in *Callinectes* and *Cancer* axons, Connor et al. (1977) first modified the Hodgkin-Huxley equations as follows to fit with the somewhat different Na^+ and K^+ currents. The sodium conductance parameters were shifted toward more positive potentials, and the activation and inactivation functions were overlapped more than in the original Hodgkin-Huxley theory. The potassium conductance parameters were also moved toward more positive potentials, and the peak potassium conductance was lowered. These changes slow and weaken the delayed potassium current to agree with that seen in crustacean axons. The model now gives a good representation of the action potential in these axons but only permits repetitive firing down to a lower limit of 77 ap per sec. When an early outward current is added to the model, it becomes fully able to duplicate the range of frequencies seen in the real axons, i.e., 2–350 ap per sec. The currents leading up to an action potential in the complete model are shown in Figure 6. I_K, I_{Na}, and I_l are the adjusted Hodgkin-Huxley potassium, sodium, and leak currents. I_A is the early outward current. I_A starts large and positive (outward), being initially opposed by I_l, and decreases slowly until the

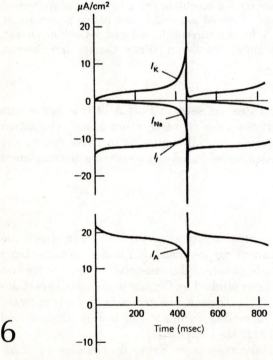

6

Ionic currents during repetitive firing in model of *Callinectes* axons. I_K, delayed potassium current; I_{Na}, inward sodium current; I_l, leak current; and I_A, early outward current. (From Connor et al., 1977.)

next spike. I_{Na} and I_K increase later in the interval. The early part of the voltage trajectory, and hence the possibility of a long interspike interval, is determined by I_A. The most important feature of this model is that it is based entirely on measured conductances and so eliminates the need for assumptions. This is a considerable advance over the application of squid-axon parameters in attempting to model completely different structures.

FREQUENCY ADAPTATION*

Adaptation, i.e., slowing of repetitive discharge in response to a maintained stimulus, is not a feature of any of the models discussed so far. Yet it is seen in many receptors and neurons and must be included in a complete model. One source of this kind of slowing in the crayfish stretch receptor is the activation of an electrogenic pump (Sokolove and Cooke, 1971). Sodium influx during the action potentials produced by a constant current causes an elevation of the intracellular Na^+ concentration. This stimulates the membrane sodium pump (see Chapter 4), producing a hyperpolarization that decreases the firing rate. The effect may be blocked by application of strophanthidin or lithium, which are known to interfere with the sodium pump. This is shown in Figure 7. Part A_1 is the normal curve of frequency versus time after the onset of a maintained step of outward current; the firing rate declines exponentially to a final level slightly more than half the initial rate. In A_2, the same step of current is applied with 1 mM strophanthidin in the bathing solution, and no adaptation is seen. A_3 shows the recovery after washing out the strophanthidin. Parts B_1–B_3 show that the same blocking of adaptation is produced when the sodium in the saline solution is replaced with lithium. This is a neat experiment, and it means that the electrogenic-pump mechanism is a sufficient explanation of adaptation in this receptor.

Connor and Stevens (1971b) mentioned a slow potassium conductance in *Anisodoris* neurons that increases following a train of spikes and that could cause slowing of repetitive discharge. Brodwick and

---

* A note on terminology: In the original use of the term "adaptation," it was the sensory receptor that adapted to the stimulus and not the associated nerve fiber (Adrian and Zotterman, 1926). Hence, adaptation had generally been considered a property of receptors and not of neurons. "Accommodation" in neurons is used to indicate an increase in threshold with a slowly rising stimulus (Solandt, 1936; Araki and Otani, 1959; Bradley and Somjen, 1961). Neurons that can fire repetitively usually show little or no accommodation (Adelman, 1956; Hagiwara and Oomura, 1958; Frank and Fuortes, 1960). In order to retain this precise definition of accommodation, it seems useful to apply "adaptation" to the slowing of the discharge rate of neurons, as well as to that of receptors (Kernell, 1965; Partridge and Stevens, 1976.)

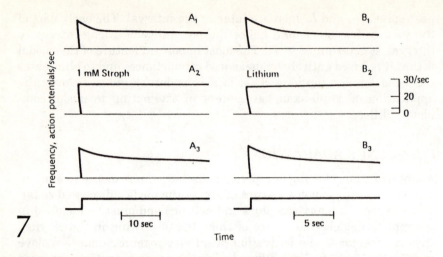

7

Blockage of frequency adaptation in crayfish stretch receptor by strophanthi-din or lithium. A_1: Frequency versus time after step-current stimulation in normal saline. A_2: Same with strophanthidin in bath. A_3: Recovery after washing out strophanthidin. B_1: Normal saline. B_2: Sodium in saline replaced with lithium. B_3: Recovery in normal saline. 5nA currents shown in bottom traces. (From Sokolove and Cooke, 1971.)

Junge (1972) found a slow K^+ conductance in the *Aplysia* R2 cell that decays with a time constant of more than 10 sec; this is about the same as the time constant for the slowing of repetitive activity in these cells. In 1976, Partridge and Stevens added a current I_s to the Connor-Stevens model of repetitive firing. I_s has the form

$$I_S = \bar{g}_s A_s(E,t)(E - E_s) \tag{10}$$

where $\bar{g}_s$ = peak slowing conductance
E_s = equilibrium potential for the slow current

and $A_s(E,t)$ satisfies the equation

$$\tau_s \frac{dA_s(E,t)}{dt} + A_s(E,t) = A_s(E,\infty) \tag{11}$$

It was not necessary to add an inactivation factor in Equation 10 to give good agreement with the slowing actually observed in these cells, although some inactivation probably does occur. The reversal potential, E_s, is quite sensitive to the external K^+ concentration, indicating that I_s is mainly a potassium current. These experiments were done at 5°C where the electrogenic sodium pump is effectively blocked, so it is not known how much the pump affects adaptation at higher temperatures. The model based on conductances alone gives a good prediction of the slowing seen in the cold.

Since calcium is known to enter molluscan cells during a burst (Gorman and Thomas, 1978), it is possible that this slow K conductance is the Ca^{2+}-activated type described in Chapter 7. However, caution must be used in making this interpretation since the application of calcium-blockers to rat pyramidal cells in vitro has been shown to block the postburst hyperpolarization but not the slowing of repetitive firing (Jones and Heinemann, 1988). The slowing may be related to a type of Ca^{2+}-induced inactivation of a calcium current (see next section).

THE BURST PATTERN OF DISCHARGE

A form of neural activity more complex than simple repetition is the production of bursts of action potentials separated by periods of inactivity. This pattern of firing is seen in many different neural structures; one example is the mammalian respiratory system, where some nerve cells fire only during inspiration or expiration. This behavior may result from an endogenous process within a single cell or it may arise from reciprocal connections in a nerve network.

Bursting was seen in *Aplysia* neurons by Tauc (1960) and Arvanitaki and Chalazonitis (1961) and is shown in Figure 8. Each burst lasts about 14 sec and consists of 23–24 spikes; the bursts are separated by about 32 sec. Following each burst, the potential is hyperpolarized by about 23 mV, then slowly returns to the threshold level. There are several reasons for thinking this pattern results from endogenous activity: (1) it may be altered by currents applied to this cell; (2) it is not interrupted by low-calcium or high-magnesium solutions, which would be expected to block any synaptic connections; (3) it has been observed in a neuron with a ligature around the axon

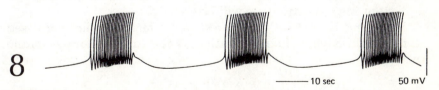

8

10 sec   50 mV

Burst discharge in *Aplysia* R15 cell. (From Strumwasser, 1965.)

(thus excluding synaptic influences from the cell body [Alving, 1968]) and in a trypsinized cell that was completely isolated from the rest of the ganglion (Chen et al., 1971).

Two principal mechanisms could cause the cessation of the burst and the following quiescent period: (1) an electrogenic pump might be activated by sodium inflow during the burst and produce the postburst hyperpolarization (Chapter 4) or (2) some membrane conductances might vary between the bursts. For instance, the potassium conductance might be large after a burst and then relax to a lower level, initiating the next burst. Evidence that the postburst hyperpolarization is not due to the activity of an electrogenic pump was presented by Gainer (1972) in the snail, *Otala* and by Carpenter (1973) and Junge and Stephens (1973) in *Aplysia*. These authors observed bursting activity in the presence of ouabain and strophanthidin and in lithium saline; all block electrogenic sodium pumps in all cases where they have been tried. Thus, in these cells, a conductance mechanism had to be sought for the production of bursts.

The only two cations with inward-directed chemical gradients (that could thus provide the depolarizing drive leading up to the burst) are sodium and calcium. There has been some argument in the literature about which of these ions is most important for bursting. Smith et al. (1975) strongly implicated sodium as the persistent inward-current carrier in *Aplysia* and *Otala*. On the other hand, Eckert and Lux (1976) concluded that the persistent current in *Helix* was carried by calcium. This may be a species difference, or it could be a result of the different voltage-clamp techniques used. In any case, given that a depolarizing drive exists in the interburst interval, a number of authors have postulated that a time-varying K conductance causes the cessation of the burst (Waziri et al., 1965; Gainer, 1972; Carpenter, 1973; Junge and Stephens, 1973). The increase in K conductance following a burst in the *Aplysia* R15 cell is probably activated by calcium, which enters during the burst (Gorman and Thomas, 1978). A convincing demonstration of larger outward current early in the interburst period was given by Carnevale (1973). It is also likely that the inward (Na^+ or Ca^{2+}) current varies during the interburst period. However, a sufficient model of burst activity can be constructed with a constant inward current, as will be seen.

Plant and Kim (1976) have presented a model of bursting based on modified Hodgkin-Huxley equations. Their equation for membrane current is

$$
\begin{aligned}
I = C\frac{dV}{dt} &+ (\bar{g}_I X_I^3 Y_I + g_T)(V_I - V) \\
&+ (\bar{g}_K X_K^4 + \bar{g}_A X_A Y_A + \bar{g}_P X_P)(V_K - V) \\
&+ g_I(V_I - V) + I_{ep}
\end{aligned}
\tag{12}
$$

where $\bar{g}_I$ = peak inward-current conductance
  g_T = persistent inward-current drive for bursting
  $\bar{g}_K$ = peak delayed K conductance
  $\bar{g}_A$ = peak transient K conductance
  $\bar{g}_P$ = peak of slow K conductance, which changes in interburst interval
  g_l = leak conductance
  I_{ep} = constant current due to electrogenic pump
  X and Y are activation and inactivation parameters

This model is different from that of Connor and Stevens (1971b) (aside from the g_T and g_P conductances) in that the activation parameter X_A is not raised to the fourth power, the equilibrium potential for the early outward current is assumed to be equal to V_K, and the electrogenic pump term is included. With a suitable choice of parameters, it gives a good representation of the normal bursting seen in the *Aplysia* R15 cell. It also predicts another finding in these cells: When TTX is added to the bathing solution, the action potentials are blocked and slow waves with the same period as the bursts are seen (Strumwasser, 1968; Mathieu and Roberge, 1971; Junge and Stephens, 1973). This is duplicated in the model simply by setting $g_I = 0$.

In the model of Plant and Kim, the slow waves, like the bursting itself, are not implied by simple knowledge of the currents giving rise to the action potential. In order to make these predictions, this model or one like it is an absolute requirement.

More recent studies with voltage-clamped bursting neurons have further dissected the currents in the interburst period. As shown in Figure 9B, from a study by Kramer and Zucker (1985), the current in *Aplysia* neurons L2–L6 may be separated into three phases. The first is a Ca^{2+}-sensitive potassium current that produces a hyperpolarization after the last action potential in the burst. The next phase (II) is a slow inward current that can be carried either by sodium or by calcium and is not strongly affected by the membrane potential. Phase III of the interburst current is an apparent outward current, but is actually caused by inactivation of a persistent inward calcium current that is always present in these neurons. (This Ca^{2+}-induced inactivation of Ca^{2+} currents has been shown previously in *Aplysia* neurons by Eckert and Tillotson [1981].) Similar results with the interburst currents in the R15 neuron were also seen by Adams and Levitan (1985). Thus, as further refinements are added to the ionic theories of burst production, better and better agreement is obtained with the experimental observations. This is part of the productive duality of theory and experiment in science.

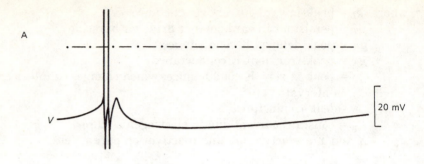

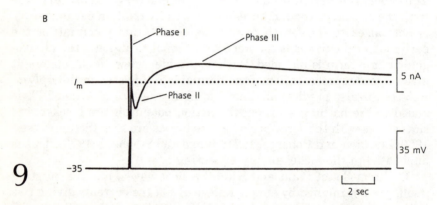

9

Potential and current during the interburst period in an *Aplysia* neuron. A: membrane potential (broken line = zero potential). B: Voltage-clamp current following a brief depolarization from about −35 mV to 0 mV. Different phases of current explained in the text. (From Kramer and Zucker, 1985.)

PROBLEMS

1. Plot the curve of frequency versus stimulus current for Adrian's model of repetitive firing, over the domain of 1–10 times minimal stimulus.

2. Plot the frequency-current curve for a model of repetitive firing in which the potential follows $V_m = IR_m(1 - e^{-t/\tau_m})$ and a spike occurs when $V_m = V_t$, a constant. Use the values $R_m = 1$ megohm, $\tau_m = 0.1$ sec, $V_t = 10$ mV, and use values of I from 10 to 100 nA.

3. For the two-factor model given in Equations 3 and 4, write an expression for I, the applied current, in terms of the time t at which the potentials V_m and V_t become equal.

4. Using intervals of t between 0.01 and 1.0 sec, find the corresponding values of I in the model of Problem 3 and plot the firing frequency versus stimulus current. Use the values $R_m = 1$ megohm, $\tau_m = 0.1$ sec, A = 0.1 mV·sec, and B = 9.0 mV.

5. In Partridge and Stevens's model of adaptation (Equations 10 and 11), after a step depolarization to -40 mV, the quantity $A_s(E,\infty)$ is approximately equal to 1 and the time constant τ_s is about 1 sec. The solution to Equation 11 is thus $A_s(-40,t) = 1 - e^{-t}$. Plot the time course of I_s for the first 5 sec following this step of potential, assuming $g_s = 1.4$ μS and $E_s = -60$ mV.

REFERENCES

Adams, W. B., and Levitan, I. B. 1985. Voltage and ion dependences of the slow currents which mediate bursting in *Aplysia* neurone R15. *J. Physiol.* 360, 69–93.

Adelman, W. J. 1956. The excitable properties of three types of motor axons. *J. Gen. Physiol.* 40, 251–262.

Adrian, E. D. 1928. *The Basis of Sensation.* New York, Hafner.

Adrian, E. D., and Gelfan, S. 1933. Rhythmic activity in skeletal muscle fibres. *J. Physiol.* 78, 271–287.

Adrian, E. D., and Zotterman, Y. 1926. The impulses produced by sensory nerve endings. *J. Physiol.* 61, 151–171.

Alving, B. O. 1968. Spontaneous activity in isolated somata of *Aplysia* pacemaker neurons. *J. Gen. Physiol.* 51, 29–45.

Alving, B. O. 1969. Differences between pacemaker and nonpacemaker neurons of *Aplysia* on voltage clamping. *J. Gen. Physiol.* 54, 512–531.

Araki, T., and Otani, T. 1959. Accommodation and local response in motoneurons of toad's spinal cord. *Jpn. J. Physiol.* 9, 69–83.

Arvanitaki, A. 1939. Recherches sur la réponse oscillatoire locale de l'axone géant isolé de «Sepia». *Arch. Int. Physiol.* 49, 209–256.

Arvanitaki, A., and Chalazonitis, N. 1961. Slow waves and associated spiking in nerve cells of *Aplysia. Bull. Inst. Oceanogr. Monaco* 58, No. 1224, 1–15.

Begenisich, T. 1975. Magnitude and location of surface charges on *Myxicola* giant axons. *J. Gen. Physiol.* 66, 47–65.

Bradley, K., and Somjen, G. G. 1961. Accommodation in motoneurones of the rat and cat. *J. Physiol.* 156, 75–92.

Brink, F. Bronk, D. W., and Larrabee, M. G. 1946. Chemical excitation of nerve. *Ann. N. Y. Acad Sci.* 47, 457–485.

Brismar, T. 1973. Effects of ionic concentration on permeability properties of nodal membrane in myelinated nerve fibres of *Xenopus laevis*. Potential clamp experiments. *Acta Physiol. Scand.* 87, 474–484.

Brodwick, M. S., and Junge, D. 1972. Post-stimulus hyperpolarization and slow potassium conductance increase in *Aplysia* giant neurone. *J. Physiol.* 223, 549–570.

Calvin, W. H. 1978. Setting the pace and pattern of discharge: do CNS neurons vary their sensitivity to external inputs via their repetitive firing processes? *Fed. Proc.* 37, 2165–2170.

Carnevale, N. T. 1973. Voltage clamp analysis of the slow oscillations in bursting neurons reveals two underlying current components, Ph. D. Dissertation, Department of Physiology, Duke University, Durham, N. C.

Carpenter, D. O. 1973. Ionic mechanisms and models of endogenous discharge of *Aplysia* neurones. *Neurobiology of Invertebrates.* J. Salancki (ed.). Budapest, Hung. Acad. Sciences, 35–58.

Carpenter, D., and Gunn, R. 1970. The dependence of pacemaker discharge of *Aplysia* neurons upon Na$^+$ and Ca^{++}. *J. Cell. Physiol.* 75, 121–128.

Chen, C. F., von Baumgarten, R., and Takeda, R. 1971. Pacemaker properties of completely isolated neurones in *Aplysia californica*. *Nature New Biol.* 233, 27–29.

Connor, J. A. 1975. Neural repetitive firing: a comparative study of membrane properties of crustacean walking leg axons. *J. Neurophysiol.* 38, 922–932.

Connor, J. A., and Stevens, C. F. 1971a. Voltage clamp studies of a transient outward membrane current in gastropod neural somata. *J. Physiol.* 213, 21–30.

Connor, J. A., and Stevens, C. F. 1971b. Prediction of repetitive firing behaviour from voltage clamp data on an isolated neurone soma. *J. Physiol.* 213, 31–53.

Connor, J. A., Walter, D., and McKown, R. 1977. Neural repetitive firing: modifications of the Hodgkin-Huxley axon suggested by experimental results from crustacean axons. *Biophys. J.* 18, 81–102.

D'Arrigo, J. S. 1973. Possible screening of surface charges on crayfish axons by polyvalent metal ions. *J. Physiol.* 231, 117–128.

Dodge, F. A. 1972. On the transduction of visual, mechanical, and chemical stimuli. *Int. J. Neurosci.* 3, 5–14.

Dudel, J., and Trautwein, W. 1958. Der Mechanismus der automatischen rhythmischen Impulsbildung der Herzmuskelfaser. *Pflügers Arch. Gesamte. Physiol. Menschen Tiere*, 267, 553–570.

Eaton, D. C. 1972. Potassium ion accumulation near a pace-making cell of *Aplysia*. *J. Physiol.* 224, 421–440.

Eckert, R., and Lux, H. D. 1976. A voltage-sensitive persistent calcium conductance in neural somata of *Helix*. *J. Physiol.* 254, 129–151.

Eckert, R., and Tillotson, D. 1981. Calcium-mediated inactivation of of the calcium conductance in caesium-loaded giant neurones of *Aplysia californica*. *J. Physiol.* 314, 265–280.

Fessard, A. 1936. *Propriétés rhythmique de la matière vivante, II*. Paris, Hermann et Cie.

FitzHugh, R. 1961. Impulses and physiological states in theoretical models of nerve membrane. *Biophys. J.* 1, 445–466.

Frank, K., and Fuortes, M. G. F. 1960. Accommodation of spinal motoneurones of cats. *Arch. Ital. Biol.* 98, 165–170.

Fuortes, M. G. F., and Mantegazzini, F. 1962. Interpretation of the repetitive firing of nerve cells. *J. Gen. Physiol.* 45, 1163–1179

Gainer, H. 1972. Electrophysiological behavior of an endogenously active neurosecretory cell. *Brain Res.* 39, 403–418.

Gorman, A. L. F., and Thomas, M. V. 1978. Changes in the intracellular concentration of free calcium ions in a pace-maker neurone, measured with the metallochromic indicator dye arsenazo III. *J. Physiol.* 275, 357–376.

Hagiwara, S., and Oomura, Y. 1958. The critical depolarization for the spike in the squid giant axon. *Jpn. J. Physiol.* 8, 234–245.

Hill, A. V. 1936. Excitation and accommodation in nerve. *Proc. R. Soc. B* 119, 305–355.

Hodgkin, A. L. 1948. The local electric changes associated with repetitive action in a non-medullated axon. *J. Physiol.* 107, 165–181.

Jones, R. S., and Heinemann, U. 1988. Verapamil blocks the afterhyperpolarization but not the spike frequency accommodation of rat CA1 pyramidal cells in vitro. *Brain Res.* 462, 367–371.

Junge, D., and Moore, G. P. 1966. Interspike-interval fluctuations in *Aplysia* pacemaker neurons. *Biophys. J.* 6, 411–434.

Junge, D., and Stephens, C. L. 1973. Cyclic variation of potassium conductance in a burst-generating neurone in *Aplysia*. *J. Physiol.* 235, 155–181.

Kernell, D. 1965. The adaptation and the relation between discharge frequency and current strength of cat lumbosacral motoneurones stimulated by long-lasting injected currents. *Acta Physiol. Scand.* 65, 65–73.

Kernell, D., and Sjöholm, H. 1973. Repetitive impulse firing: comparisons between neurone models based on "voltage clamp equations" and spinal motoneurones. *Acta Physiol. Scand.* 87, 40–56.

Kramer, R. H., and Zucker, R. S. 1985. Calcium-dependent inward current in *Aplysia* bursting pace-maker neurones. *J. Physiol.* 362, 107–130.

Mathieu, P. A., and Roberge, F. A. 1971. Characteristics of pacemaker oscillations in *Aplysia* neurons. *Can. J. Physiol. Pharmacol.* 49, 787–795.

McLaughlin, S. G. A., Szabo, G., and Eisenman, G. 1971. Divalent ions and the surface potential of charged phospholipid membranes. *J. Gen. Physiol.* 58, 667–687.

Neher, E. 1971. Two fast transient current components during voltage clamp on snail neurons. *J. Gen. Physiol.* 58, 36–53.

Neher, E., and Lux, H. D. 1971. Properties of somatic membrane patches of snail neurons under voltage clamp. *Pflügers Arch. Gesamte Physiol. Menschen Tiere*, 322, 35–38.

Neher, E., and Lux, H. D. 1973. Rapid changes of potassium concentration at the outer surface of exposed single neurons during membrane current flow. *J. Gen. Physiol.* 61, 385–399.

Partridge, L. D., and Stevens, C. F. 1976. A mechanism for spike frequency adaptation. *J. Physiol.* 256, 315–332.

Plant, R. E., and Kim, M. 1976. Mathematical description of a bursting pacemaker neuron by a modification of the Hodgkin-Huxley equations. *Biophys. J.* 16, 227–244.

Prosser, C. L. 1978. Rhythmic potentials in intestinal muscle. *Fed. Proc.* 37, 2153–2157.

Rashevsky, N. 1933. Outline of a physico-mathematical theory of excitation and inhibition. *Protoplasma* 20, 42–56.

Shapiro, B. I., and Lenherr, F. K. 1972. Increased modulation and linearity of response to constant current stimulus. *Biophys. J.* 12, 1145–1158.

Smith, T. G., Barker, J. L., and Gainer, H. 1975. Requirements for bursting pacemaker potential activity in molluscan neurones. *Nature (Lond.)* 235, 450–452.

Sokolove, P. G., and Cooke, I. M. 1971. Inhibition of impulse activity in a sensory neuron by an electrogenic pump. *J. Gen. Physiol.* 57, 125–163.

Solandt, D. Y. 1936. The measurement of "accommodation" in nerve. *Proc. R. Soc. B* 119, 355–379.

Stein, R. B. 1967. The frequency of nerve action potentials generated by applied currents. *Proc. R. Soc. B* 167, 64–86.

Strumwasser, F. 1965. The demonstration and manipulation of a circadian rhythm in a single neuron. *Circadian Clocks.* J. Aschoff (ed.). Amsterdam, North-Holland, 442–462.

Strumwasser, F. 1968. Membrane and intracellular mechanism governing endogenous activity in neurons. *Physiological and Biochemical Aspects of Nervous Integration.* F. D. Carlson (ed.). Englewood Cliffs, N. J., Prentice-Hall, 329–341.

Tauc, L. 1960. Diversité des modes d'activité des cellules nerveuses du ganglion déconnecté de l'*Aplysia*. *C. R. Soc. Biol.* 154, 17–21.

Trautwein, W., and Kassebaum, D. G. 1961. On the mechanism of spontaneous impulse generation in the pacemaker of the heart. *J. Gen. Physiol.* 45, 317–330.

Waziri, R., Frazier, W., and Kandel, E. R. 1965. Analysis of "pacemaker" activity in an identifiable burst generating neuron in *Aplysia*. *Physiologist* 8, 300.

10

SYNAPTIC TRANSMISSION

NERVE–NERVE SYNAPSES

The term SYNAPSE is attributed to Sherrington and means "joined together." It is usually applied to the point of contact between two nerve cells, although not infrequently it is applied to the neuromuscular junction. In some synapses, the method of transmission is electrical: Membrane potential changes in one cell are conducted to another via low-resistance GAP JUNCTIONS. This is a relatively fast kind of transmission, usually possible in both directions but occasionally only in the pre- to postsynaptic direction (Furshpan and Potter, 1959). In another type of synapse, a chemical transmitter is liberated by activity in the presynaptic neuron. The transmitter diffuses across a narrow cleft between the cell membranes (about 150 Å in nerve-nerve synapses and 500 Å in the neuromuscular junction) and excites the postsynaptic cell. Chemical transmission is almost always unidirectional and is somewhat slower than electrical transmission. It is much more complex, involving excitation-secretion mechanisms on the presynaptic side and receptor-channel gating on the postsynaptic membrane.

Postsynaptic nerve cells usually receive input from many presynaptic cells, sometimes thousands of them. The presence of multiple synapses means that a single neuron can act as a center of INTEGRATION of the activity in the incoming nerve fibers. For instance, a postsynaptic action potential may be produced only when a certain number of presynaptic cells fire at about the same time (spatial summation), or only when a single presynaptic cell fires several times within a certain interval (temporal summation). In synaptic INHIBITION, the activity of one cell causes a reduction of the activity in another; an inhibitory synapse may reduce the response to an excitatory input in the same cell. Excitatory and inhibitory influences may act on a postsynaptic cell, even when it is not firing action potentials, by moving the potential toward or away from the firing threshold (or changing the membrane resistance) and thus making the cell easier or harder to excite. And the response to a single synaptic input may increase with repetition (SYNAPTIC FACILITATION) or decrease with repetition (SYNAPTIC DEPRESSION). These and probably many other mechanisms for processing neural data are thus available in a single cell.

NERVE-MUSCLE SYNAPSES

With the neuromuscular junction, it is quite easy to see that a system of *amplification* must occur between the approaching nerve impulse and the large postjuctional membrane in order for transmission to take place. A gap junction, for instance, that conducted a fraction of the presynaptic current into the postsynaptic side would have no chance of depolarizing it enough to trigger an action potential. The method of amplification is basically the same in nerve-nerve and nerve-muscle junctions: Activity in the presynaptic terminal causes liberation of transmitter, which opens ionic channels in the postsynaptic membrane. The energy for the postsynaptic spike comes from the asymmetric ion distribution across the membrane, instead of from the presynaptic spike.

The physical arrangement of a neuromuscular junction is shown in Figure 1. This electron micrograph shows a cross section of the nerve terminal indented into a muscle cell and surrounded by a Schwann cell. (The actual junction is many times as long as its cross section.) The dark-looking structures at the top of the terminal are mitochondria, and the lower portion is filled with synaptic VESICLES, which contain the transmitter (in this case, acetylcholine). Heuser and Reese (1973) have shown that liberation of acetylcholine occurs by fusion of the vesicle and nerve-terminal membranes, the vesicular contents being "dumped" into the synaptic cleft. The additional membrane added from the vesicles is then recycled to make new ones. After the transmitter diffuses across the cleft, it binds to RECEPTORS in the muscle membrane and causes an increase in conductance to ions present inside and outside the cell. This leads to depolarization in the case

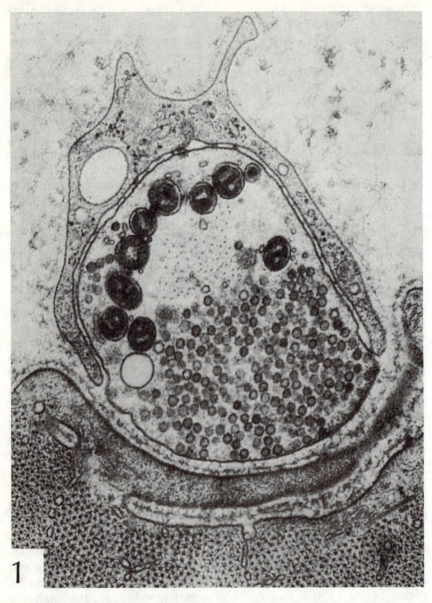

Cross section of frog neuromuscular junction. Nerve terminal indents into muscle fiber and is enclosed by Schwann cell above. Dark-staining objects are mitochondria and small structures in bottom half of terminal are synaptic vesicles. Between the terminal and the muscle endplate is the synaptic cleft; directly beneath this is an infolding of the muscle wall, the junctional fold. (Figure kindly provided by Dr. John E. Heuser.)

of an excitatory input and usually to production of an action potential in the muscle, which in turn causes contraction. The amount of transmitter that is released is either (1) bound to postsynaptic receptors, (2) hydrolyzed by enzymes such as acetylcholinesterase, or (3) taken up again by the terminal, which prevents prolonged stimulation of the receptors. All of these steps together occur in a few milliseconds.

THE POSTSYNAPTIC POTENTIAL

Quite a bit was known about synaptic transmission in 1951, the year in which the first intracellular recordings from a postsynaptic membrane were published. From focal recordings in motoneuron pools, the Eccles group in Canberra had observed extracellular synaptic potentials, as had Fatt and Katz and others using the motor endplate of frog muscle. It was understood that acetylcholine was the transmitter in the neuromuscular junction and that it acted on the postjunctional membrane to produce the endplate potential. What was lacking was the ability to measure conductance changes in postsynaptic cells and to determine which ions were involved in the production of synaptic potentials. Fatt and Katz (1951) and Brock et al. (1952) overcame this difficulty at about the same time. An intracellular recording of an excitatory postsynaptic potential (EPSP) is shown in Figure 2. The top trace is the membrane potential in a cat motoneuron, and the bottom is an extracellular recording from a spinal root containing the presynaptic fibers. A shock is delivered to the root, the compound action potential is triggered, and this in turn evokes the EPSP. The peak of the response is reached in about 1 msec, and the half-time of the decay is 2.5–3.5 msec. These authors also observed inhibitory postsynaptic potentials (IPSPs) upon stimulating presynaptic fibers from antagonist muscles (i.e., antagonistic to those whose motoneu-

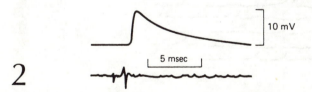

2

Excitatory postsynaptic potential (EPSP) in cat spinal motoneuron. Top trace, intracellular recording of response in postsynaptic neuron; bottom trace, extracellular recording of compound action potential in presynaptic nerve fibers. (From Brock et al., 1952.)

rons were being studied). Little was known at this point about the ionic mechanisms of the EPSP or IPSP, but, curiously, the attention of neuroscientists now began to turn toward the mechanism of release of transmitter from the presynaptic cells.

MINIATURE POSTSYNAPTIC POTENTIALS

In 1950, Fatt and Katz had tried placing an intracellular electrode directly under a motor endplate in a frog muscle. With the amplification of the recording system at a rather high level, they observed the activity shown in Figure 3. This consisted of irregularly occurring events with a mean amplitude of about 0.5 mV and a half-time of decay of about 5 msec. The mean repetition rate varied from 1 to 100 per sec between different endplates. These MINIATURE ENDPLATE POTENTIALS were not seen if the electrode was placed more than 2 mm away from an endplate. They were blocked by curare, which interferes with postsynaptic receptors for acetylcholine, and were augmented by prostigmine, an anticholinesterase. Fatt and Katz correctly attributed the MEPPs to release of small quantities of acetylcholine from isolated spots on the presynaptic terminals. In a further study (Fatt and Katz, 1952), they found that the MEPPs could not be observed in a muscle that had been previously denervated. However, spike activity in the nerve terminals was not necessary: del Castillo and Katz (1955a) later

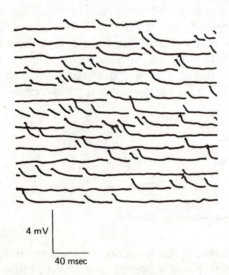

4 mV

40 msec

3

Miniature endplate potentials (MEPPs) in frog neuromuscular junction. (From Fatt and Katz, 1950.)

showed that MEPPs could be recorded in sodium-free solution in which the nervous activity coming into the terminals was presumably blocked. The miniature potentials were simply due to a random subthreshold release of acetylcholine from the nerve terminal.

In 1952, Fatt and Katz reported an observation of great functional significance: In solutions with reduced calcium concentration, the end-plate potential (EPP) evoked by nerve stimulation became very small and finally began to fail at times. When this happened, the amplitude of the endplate potentials was seen to be *quantized* in multiples of a fundamental EPP that had the same amplitude as the spontaneous miniature potentials. This is illustrated in Figure 4, which is taken

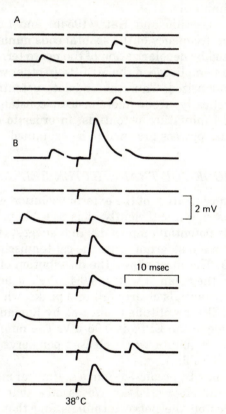

4

Spontaneous activity and evoked endplate potentials (EPPs) in the rat dia-phragm. A: Spontaneous miniature potentials. B: EPPs evoked by stimulation of phrenic nerve (stimuli applied at downward deflections) with muscle in low-calcium, high-magnesium solution. Different traces show release of 0, 1, 2, or 4 quanta. (From Liley, 1956a.)

from another preparation. Part A shows spontaneously occurring miniature potentials and Part B shows some MEPPs and evoked endplate potentials that occur with a fixed delay after the nerve stimulus (downward signals). Two of the evoked endplate potentials are the size of a single MEPP, three are twice as big, and one is four times as big. There are two failures of transmission. When a large number of evoked EPPs are studied, it can clearly be seen that the amplitudes fall in peaks that are multiples of the mean miniature-potential amplitude. The dramatic result of this seemingly odd experiment, of testing a neuromuscular junction under grossly nonphysiological conditions, is the following: The normal endplate potential is simply the sum of hundreds of miniature potentials occurring at about the same time in response to nerve stimulation.

Subsequently, del Castillo and Katz (1954b) and Liley (1956b) showed that the mean frequency of the spontaneous miniature potentials could be increased by depolarization of the nerve terminals without affecting the mean amplitude of the MEPPs. In other words, transmitter release was quantized. Thus the endplate potential could be reconstructed theoretically from more-or-less constant-amplitude "building blocks," the miniature potentials. In order to do this, the statistics of the release process first had to be examined.

PROBABILISTIC MODEL OF TRANSMITTER RELEASE

When the calcium concentration of the external solution is lowered or that of magnesium is raised sufficiently, it is possible to construct a histogram of endplate potential amplitudes that suggests that release occurs in quanta. Such a histogram, from the cat tenuissimus muscle, is shown in Figure 5. The inset shows the distribution of miniature-potential amplitudes, the mean of which is 0.4 mV. The amplitudes of the evoked endplate potentials clearly fall into peaks, which are multiples of the mean MEPP amplitude (indicated by Roman numerals). The average amplitude of the EPPs is 0.93 mV. The number of cases in which 0, 1, 2, . . . , 9 quanta were released per nerve stimulus is shown in the center of Table 1.

This distribution may be predicted from a statistical model worked out by del Castillo and Katz (1954a): We assume that there are n available release sites on the nerve terminals and that each has a probability p of releasing a quantum. Then the probability of x quanta being released by an impulse is given exactly by the binomial distribution:

$$f(x) = \frac{n_x}{N} = \frac{n!}{x!(n-x)!} p^x q^{n-x} \qquad (1)$$

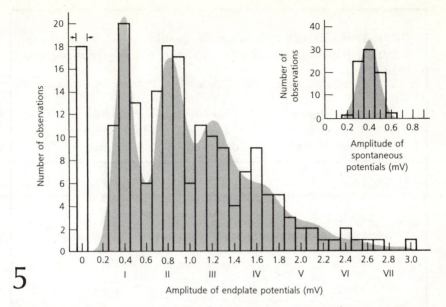

5

Quantized distribution of evoked EPP amplitudes in cat tenuissimus muscle bathed in high-magnesium solution. Left-hand peak indicates failures of transmission. Other peaks fall in multiples of the single-quantum amplitude (0.4 mV). Inset shows amplitude distribution of spontaneous miniature potentials. (From Boyd and Martin, 1956.)

where n_x = number of trials in which x quanta are released
   N = total number of trials
   p = probability of release of a single quantum
   q = probability that a quantum will not be released = $1 - p$

When the probability p becomes small and the number of available release sites large (as a rule of thumb, $p < 0.05$, $n > 100$), the binomial distribution is approximated closely by the Poisson distribution:

$$f(x) = \frac{n_x}{N} = \frac{e^{-m}m^x}{x!} \qquad (2)$$

where $m = np$ = average number of quanta released per trial.

In synaptic physiology, m is called the QUANTAL CONTENT. This distribution applies to situations in which there are many events taking place or many objects available, and a very small probability of a certain event taking place or a certain object being chosen. For

Table 1. Prediction of number of quanta released per nerve stimulation in a neuromuscular junction. (From Boyd and Martin, 1956.)

Quanta released per stimulus	No. of cases observed	Predicted by Poisson distribution
0	18	19.3
1	44	44.9
2	55	52.3
3	36	40.6
4	25	23.7
5	12	11.0
6	5	4.3
7	2	1.4
8	1	0.4
9	0	0.1

instance, in typing a printed page, many hundreds of letters are struck and there is a small probability of making a misprint each time. The number of errors per page thus follows a Poisson distribution. Similarly, whereas many telephone calls are placed in a city each day, the probability of one of these calls reaching a particular telephone is very small. Thus, the number of calls received per hour follows a Poisson distribution.

In Boyd and Martin's (1956) data, the mean number of quanta released per impulse may be estimated as follows:

$$m = \frac{\text{mean amplitude of EPPs}}{\text{mean amplitude of MEPPs}} \tag{3}$$

This yields a value of $m = 2.33$. With this value and a total of 198 stimulations, Equation 2 predicts the frequencies of release of the various numbers of quanta shown on the right side of Table 1.

The quantal content may also be calculated from the number of failures of transmission that occur in N trials: If the number of quanta released per trial follows a Poisson distribution, then

$$\frac{n_0}{N} = e^{-m} \qquad (4)$$

Thus m may be calculated as

$$m = \ln\frac{N}{n_0} \qquad (5)$$

In the above example, Equation 5 yields $m = \ln(198/18) = 2.4$. This may be taken as evidence that the release follows a Poisson distribution since it agrees well with the value found in Equation 3. These two measures of m have also been shown to remain close to each other as the rate of release with nerve stimulation is increased, by decreasing Mg^{2+} or increasing Ca^{2+} in the bathing solution (del Castillo and Katz, 1954a; Boyd and Martin, 1956). Martin (1955) has shown that for large values of release the potential effects of the quanta do not add linearly since the potential during the EPP becomes closer and closer to the equilibrium potential, and m must be estimated from

$$m = \frac{\bar{v}}{\bar{v}_1}\left(1 - \frac{\bar{v}}{V_0}\right)^{-1} \qquad (6)$$

where $\bar{v}$ = average EPP size
  $\bar{v}_1$ = average MEPP size
  V_0 = maximum possible EPP size

At very large levels of release, the Poisson distribution does not apply, and the binomial distribution must be used.

The peaks in the EPP histogram (Figure 5) overlap considerably due to the spread of amplitudes of the quanta themselves (shown in the inset). In order to reconstruct the overlapping peaks, the following procedure was used: The individual numbers of trials in which a certain number of quanta were released (n_x) were each distributed somewhat to account for the variation in size of the MEPPs. The means of the distributions were given by xv_1 (the number of quanta released times the average MEPP size) and the variances by $x\sigma^2$, where σ was the standard deviation of the MEPP amplitudes. When the resulting curves were added, the shaded curve in Figure 5 was produced.

This statistical formulation, originally presented by del Castillo and Katz (1954a), has one main result that could be obtained only by making the model: It shows that the endplate potential may be accurately reconstructed from a variable number of miniature potentials, which are identified with the release of single quanta. In addition, it can predict the effects of reduced probability of release in high-magnesium or low-calcium solutions, by lowering p. It can explain PRESYNAPTIC INHIBITION, in which the quantal content, m, is reduced by a presynaptic stimulus (Dudel and Kuffler, 1961b). However, much caution must be exercised in discussing synaptic facilitation (increase of EPP size with repetition) or depression (decrease of EPP size) in terms of the binomial/Poisson model: Brown et al. (1976) have shown that if n varies with time or p varies from one site to another, the estimates of these parameters derived from EPP amplitude histograms can be totally incorrect. A similar quantal analysis to that in the frog neuromuscular junction has been found to hold for the cat tenuissimus muscle (Boyd and Martin, 1956), the rat diaphragm (Liley, 1956a), the crayfish opener muscle (Dudel and Kuffler, 1961a), spinal motoneurons (Kuno, 1964), and the chick ciliary ganglion (Martin and Pilar, 1964).

IDENTIFICATION OF QUANTA WITH VESICLES

Vesicles in presynaptic terminals were first observed by De Robertis and Bennett (1954) and Palade and Palay (1954). In 1956, del Castillo and Katz suggested that release of one quantum of transmitter corresponded to the emptying of one vesicle into the intercellular cleft. Subsequently, other lines of evidence have related the quanta with vesicles. A fraction of subcellular particles that contains intact synaptic vesicles may be isolated with the ultracentrifuge; the presence of acetylcholine (ACh) in this fraction indicates it is associated with the vesicles (Whittaker, 1965). Also, treatment of the frog neuromuscular junction with black widow spider venom causes massive release of transmitter and simultaneously depletes the number of vesicles seen in electron micrographs of presynaptic endings (Clark et al., 1972).

The number of ACh molecules in a single quantum may be estimated by applying ACh iontophoretically to a motor endplate through a micropipette and calculating the amount of transmitter needed to produce a depolarization equal to the amplitude of one miniature potential. This was done by Krnjević and Miledi (1958) in the mammalian neuromuscular junction, with the result of several hundred thousand molecules of ACh per quantum. This was given as an upper limit since much of the transmitter expelled from the pipette may not have reached the postsynaptic receptors. Kuffler and Yoshikami (1975) have refined the method of applying the transmitter: They treated the snake neuromuscular junction with collagenase, which loosens the connective tissue around the terminal. The motor nerve could then be physically removed, exposing the presynaptic membrane to direct application of ACh. They reported a value of less than 10,000 molecules per quantum. This is supported by calculations based on the size of vesicles (about 500 Å in diameter): If the ACh inside a vesicle is assumed to be isotonic with the external body fluids (about 320 mOsm), then a single quantum should contain about 6,000 molecules of ACh.

CALCIUM AND TRANSMITTER RELEASE

It has been known since the time of Locke (1894) that calcium ions in the external solution were necessary for transmission at the neuromuscular junction. There was some question whether the lack of calcium blocked transmitter release or inactivated the postjunctional membrane. This was resolved for sympathetic ganglia in 1940 when Harvey and MacIntosh collected and assayed ACh from perfused preparations. When calcium was omitted from the perfusing solution, the release of ACh was blocked, whereas the postganglionic cells still could respond to applied transmitter. Thus, Harvey and MacIntosh correctly foretold the essentiality of external calcium for transmitter release in chemical synapses of all kinds.

The early investigators working with the neuromuscular junction were quite aware that calcium was necessary for transmission (del Castillo and Stark, 1952; del Castillo and Katz, 1954a; Boyd and Martin, 1956; Liley, 1956a) and that magnesium interfered with transmission (del Castillo and Engbaek, 1954; del Castillo and Katz, 1954a; Boyd and Martin, 1956; Liley, 1956a). In 1957 Jenkinson applied a kinetic scheme to account for the competition of calcium and magnesium, which was amplified by Dodge and Rahamimoff (1967). Figure 6A shows the dependence of EPP amplitude on $[Ca^{2+}]$ that Dodge and Rahamimoff observed. The open circles were obtained with $[Mg^{2+}] = 0.5$ mM, squares with 2.0 mM, and the solid circles with 4.0 mM. The curvature of these lines led the authors to postulate the following relationship (at low levels of Ca^{2+}-concentration):

$$\text{EPP amplitude} = A[Ca^{2+}]^f \tag{7}$$

where A and f are constants.

When the EPP amplitude was graphed against $[Ca^{2+}]$ in a double-log plot, straight lines were obtained as in Figure 6B. This showed that the power function in Equation 7 did apply; the slopes of the lines, equal to f, were about 3.8. The value f = 4 was taken as an approximation. The effect of raising external $[Mg^{2+}]$ was to decrease the EPP amplitude at all values of $[Ca^{2+}]$, by a mechanism of competitive inhibition. The fourth-power dependency of EPP amplitude

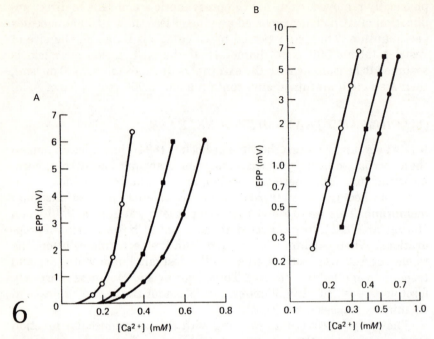

Dependence of EPP amplitude in frog muscle on Ca^{2+} concentration in the bathing solution. A: Linear plot of EPP amplitude versus Ca^{2+} concentration. B: Log (EPP amplitude) versus log (Ca^{2+} concentration). Open circles = $[Mg^{2+}]$ = 0.5 mM; squares = 2.5 mM; solid circles = 4.0 mM. (From Dodge and Rahamimoff, 1967.)

on $[Ca^{2+}]$ was consistent with the idea that four Ca^{2+} ions had to be present in a certain area of the presynaptic membrane for a quantum to be released. This was known as the COOPERATIVITY of calcium ions in transmitter release.

During the middle 1960s, Katz and Miledi carried out several more experiments in London with the frog neuromuscular junction. They showed that in preparations treated with TTX, which completely blocked the sodium channels in the presynaptic nerve, release of transmitter could still be obtained by depolarizing the terminals directly with applied currents (Katz and Miledi, 1967a). They also used the technique of filling a micropipette with concentrated CaCl₂ solution, and applying the calcium directly to the area of an endplate by removal of a negative "brake" current on the pipette (Katz and Miledi, 1965). A particularly important result obtained with this method was that, in the TTX-paralyzed preparation, focal application of calcium permitted transmitter release only if it occurred shortly before or during the depolarizing stimulus (Katz and Miledi, 1967c). This implied that calcium must normally enter the terminal exactly at the time of the presynaptic action potential. These authors also studied SYNAPTIC DELAY, or the time between the presynaptic spike and the start of the endplate potential. They found that transmitter release did not start until 1–2 msec after the end of a very brief depolarizing stimulus, and they concluded that several steps must intervene between the depolarization-induced increase in Ca^{2+} permeability and release of quanta (Katz and Miledi, 1967b).

THE SQUID SYNAPSE

One problem with the experiments on motor endplates was the lack of knowledge about the presynaptic membrane potential, which had to be an important determinant of transmitter release. The stellate synapse of the squid looked like a very good preparation to turn to for this information: Intracellular recording was possible on both pre- and postsynaptic sides (Bullock and Hagiwara, 1957), and it was apparently a chemical synapse since no electrotonic coupling could be found between the pre- and postsynaptic fibers (Hagiwara and Tasaki, 1958). Miledi and Slater (1966) carried out the straightforward experiment of removing calcium from the external solution and showing blockage of the excitatory postsynaptic potential (EPSP). Then a very interesting observation was made at about the same time by Bloedel et al. (1966), Kusano et al. (1967), and Katz and Miledi (1967d): Application of TTX to the squid synapse, which blocked the action potentials in the pre- and postsynaptic nerve fibers, did not interfere with transmitter release. When brief depolarizing pulses were applied to the presynaptic fiber through a microelectrode, EPSPs were seen that looked very much like those normally produced by nerve stimulation.

Some strong suggestions about the role of calcium in this apparently "spikeless" transmitter release in the squid were now obtained by Katz and Miledi: First they showed that by holding the presynaptic membrane potential at very positive levels near the calcium equilibrium potential (+130 mV), they could completely block the EPSP (Katz and Miledi, 1967d). A direct demonstration of calcium entry in TTX-blocked pre-terminals is given in Figure 7, from Katz and Miledi (1969). A current pulse applied to the presynaptic membrane (top trace) elicited a regenerative action potential (middle trace) that could only have been caused by entry of Ca^{2+} ions. The resulting EPSP is shown in the bottom trace. By injecting the presynaptic nerve fibers with TEA, Katz and Miledi (1969) blocked the outward K^+ current

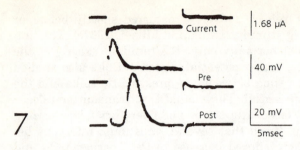

7

Regenerative action potential in presynaptic terminal of squid synapse treated with tetrodotoxin. Top: Current applied to presynaptic membrane. Middle: Presynaptic calcium spike. Bottom: EPSP in postsynaptic membrane. (After Katz and Miledi, 1969.)

occurring at the time of Ca^{2+} entry and augmented the release, shown by the size of the EPSP. All of their observations with calcium effects on different types of synapses led to the "calcium hypothesis," that entry of calcium into the presynaptic terminal is a necessary step for transmitter release. The importance of calcium for release has also been shown in the rat phrenic-diaphragm preparation (Gage and Quastel, 1966; Hubbard et al., 1968), and the crayfish neuromuscular junction (Bracho and Orkand, 1970; Ortiz and Bracho, 1972).

In 1971, Baker et al. published the first demonstration of calcium entry into nerve using the Ca^{2+}-sensitive light-emitting protein, aequorin (see Chapter 8). It was only a year later that Llinás et al. (1972) injected aequorin into a presynaptic fiber in the squid stellate synapse and obtained the result shown in Figure 8. The top trace is the current produced in a photomultiplier tube by the aequorin light signal; the solid bar in the lower line indicates a 45-sec period of repetitive stimulation of the presynaptic nerve. Following the start of

8

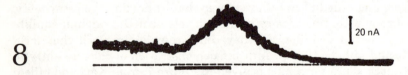

Direct demonstration of calcium entry in presynaptic terminals in squid. Terminal was injected with Ca^{2+}-sensitive photoprotein, aequorin. Top trace shows light emitted by aequorin, indicating increased Ca^{2+} concentration, during and after 45 sec of repetitive stimulation (solid bar below). (From Llinás et al., 1972.)

the stimulation, the light signal increased to more than three times the background level. This was direct evidence of calcium entry in the preterminal of the synapse.

SYNAPTIC FACILITATION

The entry of calcium into synaptic terminals has also been claimed to explain facilitation, or increase of synaptic potential size with repeated stimulation. The residual amount of calcium left over from the first synaptic event is thought to add to that from the next stimulation and augment the release of transmitter (Katz and Miledi, 1968). Charlton et al. (1982) used the Ca^{2+}-sensitive dye arsenazo III (Chapter 8) to study intracellular calcium in the squid presynaptic terminal. They found that the presynaptic Ca^{2+} concentration remained elevated for several seconds following a burst of action potentials, which would allow for a summation of residual calcium to contribute to facilitation.

Most of the earlier studies of facilitation had assumed that external calcium acted on some site near the membrane to cause transmitter release. However, more recent experiments affecting internal $[Ca^{2+}]$ make it appear that the intracellular calcium concentration is crucial in determining the rate of release (Rahamimoff et al., 1978; Augustine et al., 1987). Thus, an additional step in the process must be the diffusion of calcium ions from the Ca^{2+} channels in the membrane to the release sites. Some model studies have dealt with the details of this step (Fogelson and Zucker, 1985; Simon and Llinás, 1985). One result is that diffusion from a Ca^{2+} channel is limited approximately to the radius of a synaptic vesicle, so that two or more channels must open near a vesicle to initiate release.

PARALLEL-CONDUCTANCE MODEL OF THE POSTSYNAPTIC MEMBRANE

Most of the foregoing discussion of synapses has had to do with presynaptic mechanisms. In order to study the process by which the transmitter produces an excitatory or inhibitory response in the postsynaptic membrane, an electrical model like that in Figure 9 has been used by many authors (Fatt and Katz, 1951; del Castillo and Katz, 1955b; Coombs et al., 1955; Takeuchi and Takeuchi, 1960; Ginsborg, 1967). E_r and g_r are the resting potential and conductance of the postsynaptic membrane. E_s and g_s are the reversal potential and conductance representing the summed effects of synaptically activated channels. The capacitance has been ignored for simplicity; potential changes are assumed to occur instantaneously, although in the real

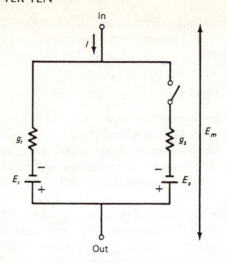

9

Electrical model of postsynaptic membrane. E_r, resting potential; g_r, resting conductance; E_s and g_s, equivalents of additional ionic channels activated by synaptic transmitter.

synapse they are slowed by the electrical properties of the membrane. The transmitter is normally regarded as activating the synaptic channels by closing the switch in Figure 9; E_m then changes from E_r to a value between E_r and E_s. For an EPSP, E_s is more positive than E_r, and for an IPSP, E_s is *usually* more negative than E_r. (Some IPSPs have reversal potentials more positive than resting, and exert their inhibitory effect by increasing the membrane conductance, thus making excitatory currents less effective in depolarizing the cell.)

When a current I is applied across the postsynaptic membrane through an intracellular microelectrode, it distributes into the resting and synaptic channels:

$$I = g_r(E_m - E_r) + g_s(E_m - E_s) \tag{8}$$

The value of potential before the synaptic stimulus is then

$$E'_m = E_r + \frac{I}{g_r} \tag{9}$$

The convention is that positive (outward) current is depolarizing. During the synaptic stimulus (after the switch is closed), the potential becomes (from Equation 8)

$$E_m = \frac{E_r g_r + E_s g_s + I}{g_r + g_s} \qquad (10)$$

The size of the postsynaptic potential is given by

$$E_m - E'_m = \frac{g_s(E_s - E_r - I/g_r)}{g_r + g_s} \qquad (11)$$

If a positive (outward) current is applied, it will reduce the size of an EPSP (make it less positive) or increase the size of an IPSP (make it more negative). It is also possible to *reverse* the direction of an IPSP by applying negative (inward) current: When $I/g_r < E_s - E_r$, the IPSP will invert and look like an EPSP. That this happens in real synapses is shown in Figure 10, which consists of data obtained from a spinal neuron by stimulation of an inhibitory afferent nerve (Coombs et al., 1955). The normal resting potential is -74 mV, and the IPSP size with no applied current is shown in D. In A–C, a depolarizing (outward) current was injected into the motoneuron through one side of a double-barreled microelectrode, causing the IPSP amplitude to increase. In E–G, hyperpolarizing (inward) current was applied, causing the IPSP to reverse near -82 mV. This behavior can be understood in terms of the model by assuming that the equilibrium potential E_s is about -82 mV and that when the postsynaptic conductance increases the membrane potential is drawn toward E_s. If the potential is held below (more negative than) E_s prior to synaptic stimulation, then the IPSP turns over.

In addition, Coombs et al. (1955) were able to change the sign of the IPSP by altering ion concentrations inside the motoneuron: Injection of Cl^- ions reversed the IPSP at potentials near resting. The effect of the injection on the model parameters was simply to make E_s more positive. Thus, E_s followed E_{Cl} (the Nernst potential for chloride), indicating that the inhibitory synaptic channels had a large amount of chloride conductance.

IONIC BASIS OF THE POSTSYNAPTIC POTENTIAL

To understand the ionic conductance changes involved in postsynaptic responses, a particularly valuable technique has been that of iontophoretic application of transmitters. This consists of filling a micropipette with a charged transmitter and placing the tip near an active synapse. The transmitter is then expelled from the pipette by a pulse of current. Under these conditions, the ionic composition of the fluid

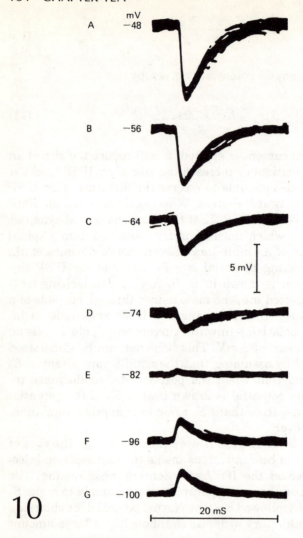

Reversal of inhibitory postsynaptic potential in a cat motoneuron by means of injected current. Outward current applied in A to C; no current in D; inward current in E to G. Values on left show potential at which membrane was held before synaptic stimulation. (From Coombs et al., 1955.)

surrounding the postsynaptic cell can be altered radically and the effects on the transmitter response examined. (Similar experiments with the neurally evoked synaptic potential are more difficult to interpret since the ionic composition of the bathing solution also affects the presynaptic fibers.)

Nastuk (1953) first used the iontophoretic technique to apply ACh in controlled amounts to a single motor endplate. Then del Castillo and Katz (1955b) showed that an amount of ACh that produced a large response when applied to the outside of the cell was completely ineffective when injected into the cell. They concluded that there were specific ACh RECEPTORS on the outer surface of the endplate membrane.

Fatt and Katz (1951) had felt that ACh acted on the postsynaptic membrane by producing a nonspecific increase in permeability to all ions present, including anions. In 1960, Takeuchi and Takeuchi varied the external chloride concentration and showed that this had no effect on the endplate potential, hence no change in the chloride conductance occurred during synaptic excitation. However, both the sodium and potassium conductances did increase, in a ratio of about $g_{Na}/g_K = 1.29$. This was very nonspecific compared to the conductance ratio of more than 10:1 seen during the squid action potential, for instance. More recent studies have shown the highly nonselective nature of the ACh receptor channel: The order of selectivities in the frog neuromuscular junction is $Tl^+ > NH_4^+ > Cs^+ > K^+, Na^+ > Li^+$ (Adams et al., 1980). This probably reflects the large diameter of the channel pore (Hille, 1992).

RECEPTORS AND CHANNELS

Since it is apparent that a transmitter such as ACh acts by binding to receptors on the outside of the postsynaptic membrane and since the effects of the transmitter are ionic channel openings, it is interesting to consider the number of receptors and channels. One very useful technique for counting the receptors has been to apply the snake venom component, α-bungarotoxin. This substance blocks neuromuscular transmission by binding irreversibly to the receptors. By labeling the toxin with tritium, it is possible to permanently mark the location of the receptors on the endplate and count them directly from autoradiographs. This method gives a total count of about 3×10^7 binding sites per endplate in mammals (Porter and Barnard, 1975). Since the area of the endplate membrane is about 3000 μm^2, this implies a density of 10^4 binding sites per μm^2. This figure has also been found for the endplate in snakes (Burden et al., 1975), and Fertuck and Saltpeter (1976) found as many as 20,000/μm^2 opposite the active zones of mouse neuromuscular junctions. Since it is possible that up to four of the five ACh receptor subunits may bind to α-bungarotoxin (Conti-Triconi and Raftery, 1982), the receptor density may be one-fourth of the above site densities, or in the neighborhood of 2500–5000/μm^2. From studies of the agonist concentration dependence of endplate conductance, apparently two ACh molecules must bind to each receptor/channel complex to cause it to change to a conductive state (Chapter 12).

MODELS OF SYNAPTIC TRANSMISSION

There is now enough quantitative data (and there are sufficient theories of mechanisms in the field of synaptic physiology) to permit the construction of models of the overall process of transmission. Several approaches have been taken to this subject, starting from very different viewpoints (Wei, 1968; Magleby and Stevens, 1972b; Llinás et al., 1976). While it is not strictly possible to select any "best" model, each demonstrates mechanisms that are possible and sufficient to explain one or more aspects of transmission.

The model of Llinás et al. (1976) was formulated to explain the relation of presynaptic and postsynaptic potentials in the squid synapse. It is based on the calcium current in the preterminal membrane, which is modeled as follows:

$$I_{Ca} = (G) \cdot j \tag{12}$$

where (G) = number of Ca^{2+} channels in the open form
j = inward current through a single open channel

(G) is considered to vary with time and potential; j depends on potential but not time. Starting from $(G) = 0$, the variation of (G) with time following a step of the presynaptic membrane potential is

$$(G) = (G)_0 \left(\frac{k_1}{k_1 + k_2} \left[1 - e^{-(k_1 + k_2)t} \right] \right)^n \tag{13}$$

where $(G)_0$ = total number of channels
k_1 and k_2 are forward and backward rate constants for formation of subunits of the channels
n = number of subunits that must be in open form for a channel to open

The single-channel current is obtained from Nernst-Planck considerations as

$$j = \frac{c_i - c_o e^{-2\epsilon V/kT}}{1 - e^{-2\epsilon V/kT}} \frac{2D\epsilon}{kT} \frac{A}{l} \cdot V \tag{14}$$

where

c_i and c_o = internal and external Ca^{2+} concentrations

ϵ = electronic charge

k = Boltzmann's constant

T = temperature, K

D = diffusion constant

A = cross-sectional area of a gate

l = thickness of the membrane

V = membrane potential

The postsynaptic potential was found to vary linearly with presynaptic (Ca^{2+}) current and to start about 200 μsec after the onset of I_{Ca}. When the presynaptic potential was varied with the model so as to reproduce an action potential, the curves shown in Figure 11 were obtained. Curve a is the time course of the Ca^{2+}-channel formation, or (G).

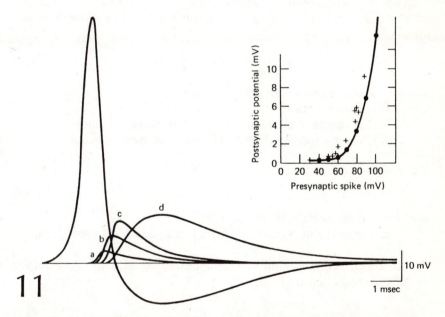

Computer model of transmission in squid synapse. Presynaptic action potential (largest deflection) shown in relation to (a) the number of calcium channels in the "open" state, (b) calcium current in presynaptic terminal, (c) current in postsynaptic membrane, and (d) postsynaptic potential. Inset shows variation of peak postsynaptic potential with peak amplitude of presynaptic spike; circles, calculated +'s, observed. (From Llinás et al., 1976.)

Curve b is I_{Ca}. Curve c is the postsynaptic current, and curve d is the postsynaptic potential. The inset shows a plot of the postsynaptic potential amplitude versus amplitude of the presynaptic spike. The solid circles define the predicted relationship and the +'s show the relationship observed in a real synapse. The best-fitting value of n in this example was 5, which can be taken to mean that each Ca^{2+} channel consists of five subunits. The model is thus able to predict the postsynaptic potential, given the time course of the presynaptic potential.

The model of Magleby and Stevens (1972b) treated some postsynaptic mechanisms in the neuromuscular junction. It was known that (1) the declining phase of the endplate currents under voltage clamp followed a simple exponential course with time constant $1/\beta$ and (2) the rate constant β varied exponentially with membrane potential (Kordaš, 1969; Magleby and Stevens, 1972a). The starting assumption for the model is that a molecule of transmitter (ligand) forms a complex with one membrane-bound receptor, opening one ionic channel in the endplate. The ligand binding and channel activation proceed as follows:

$$\text{T} + \text{R} \underset{k_2}{\overset{k_1}{\rightleftharpoons}} \text{T} \cdot \text{R} \underset{\beta}{\overset{\alpha}{\rightleftharpoons}} \text{T} \cdot \text{R}^* \tag{15}$$

where T is the transmitter, acetylcholine
 R is the receptor
 T·R is the complex associated with a closed channel
 T·R* is the complex associated with an open channel

The endplate conductance, g, is given by

$$g = \gamma x \tag{16}$$

where γ = single-channel conductance
 x = number of receptors complexed and in the "open" form

By an argument involving the distribution of ACh in the synaptic cleft, it is concluded that

$$\frac{dg}{dt} = -\beta g \tag{17}$$

where β is the rate constant for closing of channels.

And from a consideration of the effects of complexation on the dipole moment of the receptor it is found that

$$\beta(V) = \nu\, e^{-U_0/kt}\, e^{V\mu/MkT} \tag{18}$$

where ν = effective vibration frequency of the complex
     k = Boltzmann's constant
     T = temperature, K
     U_0 = free energy difference between "closed" and "open states of the complex
     μ = difference in dipole moment of the two states normal to the electric field
     M = effective thickness of the membrane
     V = membrane potential

These equations adequately describe the potential dependence of the rate constants observed in real muscles. This approach has been applied by Wathey et al. (1979) to the cholinergic junction in the electroplaque; in this case, it is assumed that two ACh molecules must bind with receptors to cause the channel to open.

LIGHT-ACTIVATED SYNAPTIC AGONISTS

Some of the most informative approaches to studying excitable membranes have involved step changes in just one variable at a time: potential steps under voltage clamp, rapid changes of external ion concentrations, temperature, or drug concentrations. Until recently, the rapidity of application of drugs was limited by the speed of exchange of bathing solutions or of diffusion of compounds from around the tip of an iontophoresis electrode. This delay has been eliminated by an elegant procedure worked out by Lester and co-workers (Nass et al., 1978): The eel electroplaque is covered with acetylcholine receptors and gives a strong depolarizing response or inward current under voltage clamp when ACh is applied to it. The cholinomimetic compound 3,3-bis(α-[trimethylammonium]methyl)azobenzene (Bis-Q) in the inactive *cis* form may be applied without effect in the solution surrounding an electroplaque. When a light flash impinges on the Bis-Q, it converts the compound to the highly potent *trans*-Bis-Q in a few microseconds. Thus the electroplaque membrane may be subjected to a "concentration step" of agonist, and the resulting changes in currents may be observed. One of the results obtained in this study is that the closing rate of the ionic channels (β, in Equation 17, above) is 100 times as fast when the agonist is in the *cis* form as when it is in the *trans* form.

Bis-Q has been applied to other preparations such as fish muscle (Weinstock, 1983), where the current during a light flash was shown to desensitize along an exponential time course. This suggested that the desensitization was produced by a first-order process. Bis-Q can even be used to study the kinetics of opening and closing of directly recorded single channels (Chabala et al., 1986). Further details of how single ACh receptor/channel mechanisms operate to produce postsynaptic potentials will be presented in Chapters 11 and 12.

PROBLEMS

1. In one of del Castillo and Katz's early experiments with frog muscle, the average EPP amplitude was 0.495 mV and the average MEPP amplitude was 0.875 mV. What was the quantal content of this synapse?

2. In the above experiment, 328 nerve stimuli were applied to test the statistics of transmitter release. If the number of quanta released per stimulus followed a Poisson distribution, how many failures of transmission would be expected?

3. In Problem 2, how many instances of simultaneous release of two quanta would be expected?

4. If a vesicle in a neuromuscular junction is 500 Å in diameter and the internal acetylcholine concentration is 160 mM, calculate the number of ACh molecules contained in the vesicle.

5. In Katz and Miledi's work with the squid synapse treated with TTX and TEA, transmission was blocked by depolarizing the presynaptic terminal to +130 mV. If this is taken as the calcium equilibrium potential and the external Ca^{2+} concentration is 11 mM, find the internal Ca^{2+} concentration.

6. The values in Figure 9 appropriate to the frog neuromuscular junction are $E_r = -90$ mV, $g_r = 5 \times 10^{-6}$ S, $E_s = -15$ mV, and $g_s = 5 \times 10^{-5}$ S. Calculate the peak amplitude of the endplate potential with no applied current.

7. According to Gage and Armstrong (1968), the additional shunt conductance added to the frog's endplate by a single miniature potential is 5.5×10^{-8} S. If the single-channel conductance is 25pS, how many channels are opened by a single quantum?

REFERENCES

Adams, D. J., Dwyer, T. M., and Hille, B. 1980. The permeability of endplate channels to monovalent and divalent metal cations. *J. Gen. Physiol.* 75, 493–510.

Augustine, G. J., Charlton, M. P., and Smith, S. J. 1987. Calcium action in transmitter release. *Annu. Rev. Neurosci.* 10, 633–693.

Baker, P. F., Hodgkin, A. L., and Ridgway, E. B. 1971. Depolarization and calcium entry in squid giant axons. *J. Physiol.* 218, 709–755.

Bloedel, J., Gage, P. W., Llinás, R., and Quastel, D. M. J. 1966. Transmitter release at the squid giant synapse in the presence of tetrodotoxin. *Nature (Lond.)* 212, 49–50.

Boyd, I. A., and Martin, A. R. 1956. The end-plate potential in mammalian muscle. *J. Physiol.* 132, 74–91.

Bracho, H., and Orkand, R. K. 1970. Effect of calcium on excitatory neuromuscular transmission in the crayfish. *J. Physiol.* 206, 61–71.

Brock, L. G., Coombs, J. S., and Eccles, J. C. 1952. The recording of potentials from motoneurones with an intracellular electrode. *J. Physiol.* 117, 431–460.

Brown, T. H., Perkel, D. H., and Feldman, M. W. 1976. Evoked neurotransmitter release: statistical effects of nonuniformity and nonstationarity. *Proc. Natl. Acad. Sci. USA* 73, 2913–2917.

Bullock, T. H., and Hagiwara, S. 1957. Intracelllular recording from the giant synapse of the squid. *J. Gen. Physiol.* 20, 565–577.

Burden, S., Hartzell, H. C., and Yoshikami, D. 1975. Acetylcholine receptors at neuromuscular synapses: phylogenetic differences detected by snake α-neurotoxins. *Proc. Natl. Acad. Sci. USA* 72, 3245–3249.

Chabala, L. D., Gurney, A. M., and Lester, H. A. 1986. Dose-response of acetylcholine receptor channels opened by a flash-activated agonist in voltage-clamped rat myoballs. *J. Physiol.* 371, 407–433.

Charlton, M. P., Smith, S. J., and Zucker, R. S. 1982. Role of presynaptic calcium ions and channels in synaptic facilitation and depression at the squid giant synapse. *J. Physiol.* 323, 173–193.

Clark, A. W., Hurlbut, W. P., and Mauro, A. 1972. Changes in the fine structure of the neuromuscular junction of the frog caused by Black Widow Spider venom. *J. Cell. Biol.* 52, 1–14.

Conti-Triconi, B. M., and Raftery, M. A. 1982. The nicotinic cholinergic receptor: correlation of molecular structure with functional properties. *Annu. Rev. Biochem.* 51, 491–530.

Coombs, J. S., Eccles, J. C., and Fatt, P. 1955. The specific ionic conductances and the ionic movements across the motoneuronal membrane that produce the inhibitory post-synaptic potential. *J. Physiol.* 130, 326–373.

del Castillo, J., and Engbaek, L. 1954. The nature of the neuromuscular block produced by magnesium. *J. Physiol.* 124, 370–384.

del Castillo, J., and Katz, B. 1954a. Quantal components of the end-plate potential. *J. Physiol.* 124, 560–573.

del Castillo, J., and Katz, B. 1954b. Changes in end-plate activity produced by pre-synaptic polarization. *J. Physiol.* 124, 586–604.

del Castillo, J., and Katz, B. 1955a. Local activity at a depolarized nerve-muscle junction. *J. Physiol.* 128, 396–411.

del Castillo, J., and Katz, B. 1955b. On the localization of acetylcholine receptors. *J. Physiol.* 128, 157–181.

del Castillo, J., and Katz, B. 1956. Biophysical aspects of neuromuscular transmission. *Prog. Biophys.* 6, 121–170.

del Castillo, J., and Stark, L. 1952. The effect of calcium ions on the motor end-plate potentials. *J. Physiol.* 116, 507–515.

De Robertis, E., and Bennett, H. S. 1954. Submicroscopic vesicular component in the synapse. *Fed. Proc.* 13, 38.

Dodge, F. A., and Rahamimoff, R. 1967. Co-operative action of calcium ions in transmitter release at the neuromuscular junction. *J. Physiol.* 193, 419–432.

Dudel, J., and Kuffler, S. 1961a. The quantal nature of transmission and spontaneous miniature potentials at the crayfish neuromuscular junction. *J. Physiol.* 155, 514–529.

Dudel, J., and Kuffler, S. 1961b. Presynaptic inhibition at the crayfish neuromuscular junction. *J. Physiol.* 155, 543–562.

Fatt, P., and Katz, B. 1950. Some observations on biological noise. *Nature (Lond.)* 166, 597–598.

Fatt, P., and Katz, B. 1951. An analysis of the end-plate potential recorded with an intra-cellular electrode. *J. Physiol.* 115, 320–370.

Fatt, P., and Katz, B. 1952. Spontaneous subthreshold activity at motor nerve endings. *J. Physiol.* 117, 109–128.

Fertuck, H. C., and Saltpeter, M. M. 1976. Quantitation of junctional and extrajunctional acetylcholine receptors by electron microscopic autoradiography after ^{125}I-α-bungarotoxin binding at mouse neuromuscular junctions. *J. Cell Biol.* 69, 144–158.

Fogelson, A. L., and Zucker, R. S. 1985. Presynaptic calcium diffusion from various arrays of single channels: implications for transmitter release and synaptic facilitation. *Biophys. J.* 48, 1003–1017.

Furshpan, E. J., and Potter, D. D. 1959. Transmission at the giant synapses of the crayfish. *J. Physiol.* 145, 289–325.

Gage, P. W., and Armstrong, C. M. 1968. Miniature end-plate currents in voltage-clamped muscle fibre. *Nature (Lond.)* 218, 363–365.

Gage, P. W., and Quastel, D. M. J. 1966. Competition between sodium and calcium ions in transmitter release at a mammalian neuromuscular junction. *J. Physiol.* 185, 95–123.

Ginsborg, B. L. 1967. Ion movements in junctional transmission. *Pharmacol. Rev.* 19, 289–316.

Hagiwara, S., and Tasaki, I. 1958. A study on the mechanism of impulse transmission across the giant synapse of the squid. *J. Physiol.* 143, 114–137.

Harvey, A. M., and MacIntosh, F. C. 1940. Calcium and synaptic transmission in a sympathetic ganglion. *J. Physiol.* 97, 408–416.

Heuser, J. E., and Reese, T. S. 1973. Evidence for recycling of synaptic vesicle membrane during transmitter release at the frog neuromuscular junction. *J. Cell Biol.* 57, 315–344.

Hille, B. 1992. *Ionic Channels of Excitable Membranes*, 2nd Ed. Sunderland, Mass., Sinauer.

Hubbard, J. I., Jones, S. F., and Landau, E. M. 1968. On the mechanism by which calcium and magnesium affect the spontaneous release of transmitter from mammalian motor nerve terminals. *J. Physiol.* 194, 355–380.

Jenkinson, D. H. 1957. The nature of the antagonism between calcium and magnesium ions at the neuromuscular junction. *J. Physiol.* 138, 434–444.

Katz, B., and Miledi, R. 1965. The effect of calcium on acetylcholine release from motor nerve terminals. *Proc. R. Soc. B* 161, 496–503.

Katz, B., and Miledi, R. 1967a. Tetrodotoxin and neuromuscular transmission. *Proc. R. Soc. B* 167, 8–22.

Katz, B., and Miledi, R. 1967b. The release of acetylcholine from nerve endings by graded electric pulses. *Proc. R. Soc. B* 167, 23–38.

Katz, B., and Miledi, R. 1967c. The timing of calcium action during neuromuscular transmission. *J. Physiol.* 189, 535–544.

Katz, B., and Miledi, R. 1967d. A study of synaptic transmission in the absence of nerve impulses. *J. Physiol.* 192, 407–436.

Katz, B., and Miledi, R. 1968. The role of calcium in neuromuscular facilitation. *J. Physiol.* 195, 481–492.

Katz, B., and Miledi, R. 1969. Tetrodotoxin-resistant electric activity in presynaptic terminals. *J. Physiol.* 203, 459–487.

Kordaš, M. 1969. The effect of membrane polarization on the time course of the end-plate current in frog sartorius muscle. *J. Physiol.* 204, 493–502.

Krnjević, K., and Miledi, R. 1958. Acetylcholine in mammalian neuromuscular transmission. *Nature (Lond.)* 182, 805–806.

Kuffler, S. W., and Yoshikami, D. 1975. The number of transmitter molecules in a quantum: an estimate from iontophoretic application of acetylcholine at the neuromuscular synapse. *J. Physiol.* 251, 465–482.

Kuno, M. 1964. Quantal components of excitatory synaptic potentials in spinal motoneurones. *J. Physiol.* 1757, 81–99.

Kusano, K., Livengood, D. R., and Werman, R. 1967. Correlation of transmitter release with membrane properties of the presynaptic fiber of the squid giant synapse. *J. Gen. Physiol.* 50, 2579–2601.

Liley, A. W. 1956a. The quantal components of the mammalian end-plate potential. *J. Physiol.* 133, 571–587.

Liley, A. W. 1956b. The effects of presynaptic polarization on the spontaneous activity at the mammalian neuromuscular junction. *J. Physiol.* 134, 427–443.

Llinás, R., Blinks, J. R., and Nicholson, C. 1972. Calcium transient in presynaptic terminal of squid giant synapse: detection with aequorin. *Science* 176, 1127–1129.

Llinás, R., Steinberg, I. Z., and Walton, K. 1976. Presynaptic calcium currents and their relation to synaptic transmission: voltage clamp study in squid giant synapse and theoretical model for the calcium gate. *Proc. Natl. Acad. Sci. USA* 73, 2918–2922.

Locke, F. S. 1894. Notiz über den Einfluss physiologischer Kochsalzlösung auf die elektrische Erregbarkeit von Muskel und Nerv. *Zentralbl. Physiol.* 8, 166–167.

Magleby, K. L., and Stevens, C. F. 1972a. The effect of voltage on the time course of endplate currents. *J. Physiol.* 223, 151–171.

Magleby, K. L., and Stevens, C. F. 1972b. A quantitative description of endplate currents. *J. Physiol.* 223, 173–197.

Martin, A. R. 1955. A further study of the statistical composition of the end-plate potential. *J. Physiol.* 130, 114–122.

Martin, A. R., and Pilar, G. 1964. Quantal components of the synaptic potential in the ciliary ganglion of the chick. *J. Physiol.* 175, 1–16.

Miledi, R., and Slater, C. R. 1966. The action of calcium on neuronal synapses in the squid. *J. Physiol.* 184, 473–498.

Nass, M. M., Lester, H. A., and Krouse, M. E. 1978. Response of acetylcholine receptors to photoisomerizations of bound agonist molecules. *Biophys. J.* 24, 135–160.

Nastuk, W. L. 1953. Membrane potential changes at a single muscle end-plate produced by transitory application of acetylcholine with an electrically controlled microjet. *Fed. Proc.* 12, 102.

Ortiz, C. L., and Bracho, H. 1972. Effect of reduced calcium on excitatory transmitter release at the crayfish neuromuscular junction. *Comp. Biochem. Physiol.* 41A, 805–812.

Palade, G. E., and Palay, S. L. 1954. Electron microscopic observations of interneuronal and neuromuscular synapses. *Anat. Rec.* 118, 335–336.

Porter, C. W., and Barnard, E. A. 1975. The density of cholinergic receptors at the endplate postsynaptic membrane: ultrastructural studies in two mammalian species. *J. Membr. Biol.* 20, 31–49.

Rahamimoff, R., Erulkar, S. D., Lev-Tov, A., and Meiri, H. 1978. Intracellullar and extracellular calcium ions in transmitter release at the neuromuscular synapse. *Ann. N. Y. Acad. Sci.* 307, 583–598.

Simon, S. M., and Llinás, R. R. 1985. Compartmentalization of the submembrane calcium activity during calcium influx and its significance in transmitter release. *Biophys. J.* 48, 485–498.

Takeuchi, A., and Takeuchi, N. 1960. On the permeability of end-plate membrane during the action of transmitter. *J. Physiol.* 154, 52–67.

Wathey, J. C., Nass, M. M., and Lester, H. A. 1979. Numerical reconstruction of the quantal event at nicotinic synapses. *Biophys. J.* 27, 145–164.

Wei, L. Y. 1968. Electric dipole theory of chemical synaptic transmission. *Biophys. J.* 8, 396–414.

Weinstock, M. M. 1983. Activation and desensitization of acetylcholine receptors in fish muscle with a photoisomerizable agonist. *J. Physiol.* 338, 423–433.

Whittaker, V. P. 1965. The application of subcellular fractionation techniques to the study of brain function. *Prog. Biophys. Mol. Biol.* 15, 39–96.

11

SINGLE-CHANNEL CURRENTS IN EXCITABLE MEMBRANES

The studies by Hodgkin, Huxley and others covered in Chapters 5–7 described large-scale, or macroscopic, currents in nerve membranes. It was known that these currents must be carried by much smaller events, but the nature of these microscopic processes of excitation was unclear. Possibly the currents were carried across the membrane one ion at a time, in a continuously graded stream; or, on the other hand, some pores or "channels" might open briefly and admit thousands of ions at once. The answer came somewhat indirectly, from studies of fluctuations of potential and current in nerve and muscle membranes, and from currents recorded in artificial systems.

NOISE ANALYSIS

In the 1960s, a group in Holland was studying potential fluctuations in the frog node of Ranvier, from the standpoint of their effects on sensory coding, such as decreasing the precision of timing of neuronal discharges (Verveen, 1962, Verveen and Derksen, 1965). This preparation was a logical choice for noise studies since the small area and high resistance of the node acted to increase the potential changes resulting from any changes in transmembrane current. Low-noise amplifiers were needed for these measurements since the potential fluctuations were only a few microvolts in amplitude.

One way to characterize noise of this type is to determine the SPECTRAL DENSITY FUNCTION of the signal. This was originally done with tuned filters, which transmitted activity only in a certain small range of frequencies. The signal power present in the output of each filter then gave the distribution of power as a function of frequency. Nowadays, however, the spectral density function is usually computed as the square of the magnitude of the Fourier transform of the signal. For a pure sinusoid, all of the power is concentrated at one frequency, so the spectral density function is an impulse. For the thermal noise (or Johnson noise) in an ideal resistor, there is an equal amount of power at all frequencies, and the spectral density is given by

$$S_V(f) = 4kTR \qquad (1)$$

where $S_V(f)$ = power per Hz in voltage signal
k = Boltzmann's constant
T = temperature, K
R = resistance

This is called "white" noise since it contains all "colors," or frequencies, of signal.

In the node of Ranvier, however, Verveen and Derksen (1965) found a completely different type of noise spectrum. This is shown in Figure 1, which is a double-log plot of the square of potential/Hz (proportional to power) versus ω (equal to $2\pi \times$ frequency, f). From the straight-line relation observed, it may be concluded that

$$P \propto V^2 = Kf^{-1} \qquad (2)$$

where P = power, proportional to V^2, per unit frequency
K = a constant

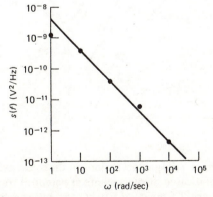

1 Spectral density function of voltage fluctuations in the node of Ranvier. Logarithm of square of potential (proportional to power) per unit frequency plotted versus logarithm of angular frequency ($=2\pi f$). (From Verveen and Derksen, 1965.)

Hence this is called "1/f" noise (sometimes "flicker" noise). It is seen in nonequilibrium systems such as semiconductors (Spangenberg, 1957), small openings between conductive solutions (Hooge and Gaal, 1970), and artificial membranes (DeFelice and Michalides, 1972).

This spectral characteristic was interesting and was not seen with linear RC circuits such as the model in Figure 2, Chapter 2. Then, in 1966, Derksen and Verveen discovered that when the node was bathed with isotonic KCl, the 1/f noise entirely disappeared, leaving only a white-noise spectrum. When Verveen et al. (1967) applied artificial currents to the membrane, the noise signal was smallest when the potential was held near E_K, the potassium equilibrium potential. These experiments suggest that 1/f noise arises from passive movement of potassium across the membrane. Poussart (1971) found cur-

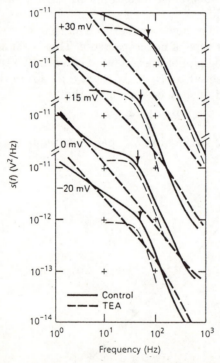

2

Spectral density functions of voltage fluctuations in the squid axon. Solid lines are spectra obtained at indicated displacements of potential from the resting level. Interrupted lines are 1/f noise seen when axons were perfused with solutions containing 50 mM TEA. Dashed lines are differences between spectra with and without TEA; these have the shape of Lorentzian functions with corner frequencies indicated by arrows. (From Fishman, 1973.)

rent fluctuations in the voltage-clamped lobster axon with the same type of spectral density function and also related the noise amplitude to potassium current.

Siebenga and Verveen (1972) looked at potential fluctuations in the node of Ranvier at more positive potentials (up to +40 mV) and observed a component of the spectral density function with the form

$$S'(f) = \frac{c}{1 + (f/f_c)^2} \tag{3}$$

where c = a constant
       f_c = "corner" frequency at which $S'(f) = c/2$

This function is called a LORENTZIAN, as it has the same form as an expression derived by Lorentz for the absorption of energy by harmonic oscillators. It was later shown (Siebenga et al., 1974) that this component of the spectrum is reduced with application of TEA but not of TTX. Hence it appears that the Lorentzian noise is produced by the opening and closing of active (delayed rectifier) K^+ channels.

With conventional intracellular electrodes of the type used by Hodgkin and Huxley, it was impossible to observe any noise fluctuations in the squid axon, due to its large surface area and low membrane resistance. This difficulty was overcome in 1973 by Fishman, who used an external "patch" electrode to isolate a small area of membrane in which potentials and currents were independent of those in the surrounding membrane. With this preparation he observed a combination of $1/f$ and Lorentzian noise in the fluctuations of potential, as shown in Figure 2. The solid lines are power spectra observed at different displacements of the membrane potential from the resting level. The heavy dashed lines show $1/f$ noise observed at each potential after the axon was perfused with 50 mM TEA. The lighter dashed lines are the differences between the spectra with and without TEA and have the form of Lorentzians (Equation 3). Thus, the entire voltage noise spectrum in these membranes can be represented by

$$S_V(f) = a + \frac{b}{f} + \frac{c}{1 + (f/f_c)^2} \tag{4}$$

where a, b, and c are the appropriate coefficients for the white, $1/f$, and Lorentzian noise.

In 1975, Fishman et al. found that the Lorentzian component disappeared when the squid axon was perfused with 100 mM cesium ions or when the internal K^+ concentration was reduced below 100 mM

with isotonic substitution of sucrose. The results and the TEA effect support the idea that Lorentzian noise is due to the opening and closing of K^+ channels. (Note that, as yet, no one had come up with a crucial test of whether channel openings were discrete or continuous, or what their amplitude and time course might be.)

MOTOR ENDPLATES

About the same time as these investigators were increasing the gain of their amplifiers and looking at membrane noise, Katz and Miledi (1971) published some observations on the excess noise produced in muscle endplates by continuous application of acetylcholine (ACh); this was interpreted in detail in a 1972 paper. Katz and Miledi recognized that the spectral density function for the voltage fluctuations was reduced at high frequencies by the electrical properties of the membrane. Accordingly, they used focal extracellular electrodes, which produced a large increase in the power at high frequencies compared to that seen with intracellular electrodes.

These investigators did not assume that a step change in conductance was produced by the interaction of synaptic transmitter and receptor. Instead, they assumed that the microscopic change in potential had the form

$$f(t) = ae^{-t/\tau} \tag{5}$$

where τ was taken as the time constant of decay of the MEPP.

The mean response, V, to a pulse of ACh could then be calculated from Campbell's Theorem (Rice, 1944) as

$$V = n \int_0^\infty f(t)dt = na\tau \tag{6}$$

where n = average frequency of channel openings.

The noise variance was given by

$$\sigma^2 = n \int_0^\infty f^2(t)dt = \frac{na^2\tau}{2} \tag{7}$$

From Equations 6 and 7,

$$\sigma^2 = \frac{Va}{2} \tag{8}$$

For an amount of ACh which gave a V of 10 mV, it was observed that the standard deviation of the noise around V was 30–50 μV. From Equation 8, the initial amplitude of the elementary event, α, may be calculated as 0.18–0.5 μV. If τ is taken as 10 msec for frog muscle, then the frequency n is given by $V/\alpha\tau$, or $2–5.6 \times 10^6$ channel openings/ sec. In this paper, they reported that the value of τ with carbachol stimulation was less than that with ACh. In a subsequent study (Katz and Miledi, 1973), they found that values of τ for decamethonium and acetylthiocholine were much smaller than that for ACh and that the value for suberyldicholine was almost twice as large as that for ACh. Evidently, the duration of channel openings was dependent on the nature of the chemical stimulus.

Anderson and Stevens (1973) managed to eliminate the problem of filtering of noise signals by the endplate membrane by means of the voltage clamp. The resulting endplate current fluctuations typically had spectral density functions such as that shown in Figure 3. The dots are the measured power at each frequency, and the solid line is a theoretical density function from a model that will be discussed in the next chapter. This function has the shape

$$S_I(f) = \frac{S_I(0)}{1 + (f/f_c)^2} \tag{9}$$

where $S_I(0)$ = the value of $S_I(f)$ at zero frequency
f_c = the "corner" frequency at which $S_I(f) = S_I(0)/2$

(A similar spectral density function was reported by Katz and Miledi in 1972.) In other words, the spectrum of current fluctuations at this potential (-60 mV) has the form of a Lorentzian.

Anderson and Stevens interpreted the endplate noise as being due to the opening and closing of varying numbers of channels, all having about the same conductance, for varying lengths of time. Unlike Katz and Miledi, they assumed that the microscopic currents turned on and off suddenly as the channels opened and closed. This model was surprisingly prophetic and received a powerful confirmation when quantized conductance changes were measured directly in muscle membranes (Neher and Sakmann, 1976).

ARTIFICIAL MEMBRANES

No doubt a strong suggestion of the quantized conductance model of nerve and muscle currents came from work with artificial membrane systems. These consisted of a lipid bilayer spread across a small hole separating two conductive solutions; different substances could then

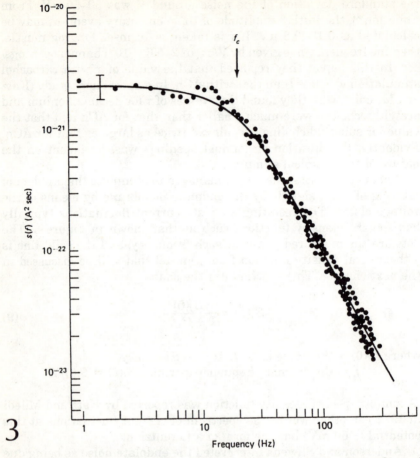

3

Spectral density function of current fluctuations produced in voltage-clamped motor endplate by continuous application of ACh. Dots are the measured power/frequency at each frequency, and the continuous curve is a theoretical density function. Error bar = ±1 SD of the current signal. f_c = corner or half-power frequency. (From Anderson and Stevens, 1973.)

be added to the bilayer and the resulting changes in membrane conductivity studied. When an extract of the bacteria *Aerobacter cloacae* was added, the membranes displayed the property of excitability, that is, they could produce action potentials similar in form to those observed in squid axons (Mueller and Rudin, 1963, 1968). The extract was named EIM, or excitability inducing material.

These artificially produced excitable systems were studied under carefully controlled conditions, including voltage clamp and high amplification, where the unitary events underlying the excitability could be dissected out. Bean et al. (1969) showed that, as the EIM was added to the membrane, the conductance increased in discrete steps, suggesting the formation of individual channels. Ehrenstein et al. (1970) found that the channels had two distinct conductance states, open and closed, and followed Ohm's law when open. The number of channels open at any time was a function of the transmembrane potential.

Discrete steps of current were also seen in bilayers when certain antibiotics were added to the membranes. Figure 4 shows currents seen with gramicidin A (Hladky and Haydon, 1970). A step of current occurs when two gramicidin molecules oppose end-to-end, forming an ion channel. The current steps add together when two or more channels are formed during a short period; the mean channel open time increases with depolarization. Similar quantized steps of current are seen with the antibiotic alamethicin (Eisenberg et al., 1973). The additive properties of the various channel types differ, however; whereas the EIM channel has only two conductance states, the alamethicin channel has up to seven!

This work with lipid bilayers was very exciting to biophysicists, as it indicated a mechanism for ion fluxes in biological membranes. The currents responsible for action potentials could be explained by the opening and closing of single ion channels in the membrane. It required a leap of faith to believe that the same mechanisms could operate in living muscle or nerve cells, but the next developments in electrophysiology showed this to be not so much a conjecture as an almost universal finding.

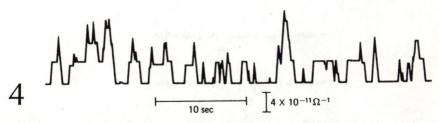

4

10 sec $4 \times 10^{-11} \Omega^{-1}$

Quantized steps of current in artificial membrane containing gramicidin. Membrane formed from glycerol monooleate in *n*-decane. Single steps of current due to formation of single ionic channels. (From Hladky and Haydon, 1970.)

SINGLE-CHANNEL RECORDING

The first major advance in observing single steps of current in a biological membrane as channels opened and closed was made by Neher and Sakmann in 1976: They took advantage of the fact that 6–10 weeks after the motor nerve is cut, muscle cells develop a widespread sensitivity to applied transmitters. These EXTRAJUNCTIONAL RECEPTORS are less densely distributed than those under the endplate. To record the activity of a small group of receptors and channels, a glass micropipette with a tip about 1 μm in diameter was filled with suberyldicholine and pressed against the muscle membrane. When the membrane potential was clamped at constant values, the currents shown in Figure 5 were recorded through the patch pipette; this method became known as the PATCH CLAMP technique. These discrete steps of current presumably represented the opening and closing of ion channels under the pipette tip; the mean channel conductance was 22 pS. The average duration of the current steps was dependent on the potential, varying e-fold for an 80-mV change.

This striking demonstration of discrete channel opening and closing in a biological membrane lent considerable validity to the preceding studies with artificial membranes and caused a profound change in the direction of work in most electrophysiology laboratories in the world. The ability to study molecular events such as single-channel

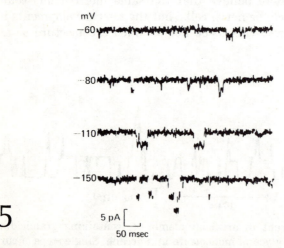

5

Discrete current steps in chronically denervated frog skeletal muscle treated with suberyldicholine. Membrane potentials indicated on left. (From Neher and Stevens, 1977.)

currents opened a new and more basic dimension for understanding membrane functions.

The next development with the patch clamp consisted of a two-orders-of-magnitude increase in the "leakage" resistance around the tip of the pipette. This resistance might amount to 200 MΩ or so when the tip was pressed against the excitable cell. By using specially cleaned pipette tips and applying slight suction, it could be increased to over 50 GΩ, or 5×10^{10} Ω. This was named the GIGOHM SEAL or GIGASEAL technique. It produced a large increase in the signal-to-noise ratio of the recording systems, so that single-channel currents could be seen much more clearly.

Figure 6 shows some modifications of the patch clamp technique, including some where the patch is physically removed from the rest of the cell membrane. The cell-attached, or "on-cell," method was the one used in the early studies of single channels. By applying suction, the membrane under the pipette can be ruptured, and a low-resistance path to the cytoplasm created. This "whole-cell" preparation can be used to voltage-clamp smaller structures. The gigaseal between the pipette tip and cell membrane is electrically tight and also physically strong. By pulling the pipette slowly away from the cell, a vesicle can be formed as shown on the left. Breaking the outer membrane then leads to the formation of an "inside-out" patch, where the cytoplasmic side is accessible for changing ionic or other chemical conditions. If the pipette is slowly withdrawn from the whole-cell preparation as on the right, some of the membrane stretches out to form an "outside-out" patch. Here, one may easily study the effects of changing external ion or drug concentrations. For more details on various patch-clamp methods, see the paper by Hamill et al. (1981) or the book by Sakmann and Neher (1983).

POTASSIUM CHANNELS

Since the acetylcholine receptor channel had been studied in muscle cells by Neher and Sakmann, above, it was natural for biophysicists to look for similar channels that might carry Na^+ and K^+ currents in nerve membranes. Conti and Neher succeeded in recording single-channel potassium currents in the squid giant axon in 1980. They inserted an L-shaped pipette into one end of the axon and pressed the tip against the inside of the membrane (an intracellular version of the on-cell method used by Neher and Sakmann), and obtained recordings such as those in Figure 7. The sodium current was blocked with external tetrodotoxin, and the steps of current seen were due to opening and closing of potassium channels. The membrane potential was

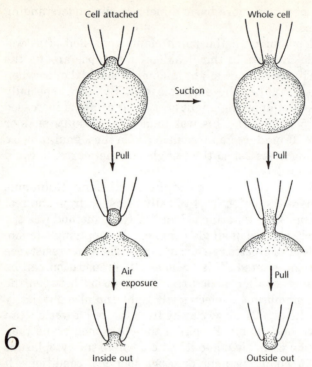

6

Patch-clamp techniques. In the cell-attached method, slight suction is applied to improve the seal between the pipette and the membrane. Increasing the suction causes the membrane under the pipette to break, creating a low-resistance path to the cell interior. By pulling the pipette away from the cell, either a vesicle (left) or a cytoplasmic bridge (right) can be formed. Exposing the vesicle to air or low-Ca^{2+} solution causes the outer membrane to break, forming an "inside-out" patch. The cytoplasmic bridge may also break, reseal at the end, and form an "outside-out" patch. Currents may then be recorded in these excised patches, which contain only a few functional channels.

held at -25 mV in A and -35 mV in B. The elementary events looked like widely spaced pulses of current with short interruptions, indicating a complex gating mechanism. The mean open time was 3.5 msec and the channel conductance was 17.5 pS, although that value was probably higher than in the living animal, due to the unusual K^+ concentrations used. This study showed that the probability of channels being in the open state increased when the membrane was depolarized, exactly as would be required to explain activation of the macroscopic K^+ current.

Other types of potassium current have also been studied with the

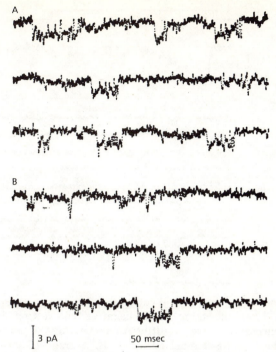

7

| 3 pA   50 msec

Single potassium-channel currents in squid axon. A was recorded at -25 mV membrane potential; B at -35 mV. Short interruptions in the pulses indicate complex gating mechanism. (From Conti and Neher, 1980.)

patch clamp technique, including transient, or A currents (Cooper and Shrier, 1985) and calcium-activated potassium currents (Barrett et al., 1982; Ewald et al., 1985).

SODIUM CHANNELS

The first successful recording of sodium-channel currents was accomplished by Sigworth and Neher (1980), in spherical structures called "myoballs" made from fused fetal muscle cells. The on-cell method of recording was used, with suction applied to the pipette to produce a gigaseal, greatly improving the current resolution. When depolarizing steps of potential were applied to the myoball membrane, the currents under the patch pipette looked like the traces in Figure 8C. Single-channel currents of constant amplitude but varying durations were seen; in some cases no channel openings occurred. When 300 such traces were added and averaged, the record shown in B was observed;

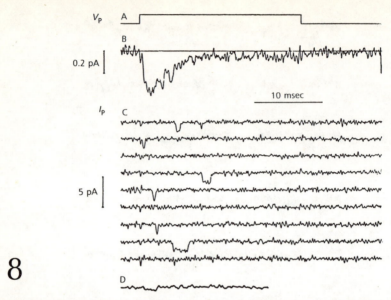

8

Single sodium-channel currents in cultured rat muscle preparation. A: Membrane potential held at −30 mV more negative than resting, depolarized by 40 mV. C: Nine current traces resulting from repeating the above depolarizing step; some show single-channel openings. B: Average of 300 such current records, showing how single-channel currents add to produce macroscopic current. D: Reduction of currents by replacing 2/3 of sodium in external medium with tetramethylammonium. (From Sigworth and Neher, 1980.)

this ENSEMBLE AVERAGE had exactly the same time course as the macroscopic sodium current in the whole membrane. When two-thirds of the external sodium was removed, the currents were reduced almost to zero (D). Thus, the identity of the summed single-channel currents with the whole-membrane Na^+ current was demonstrated. The mean open time for these channels was 0.7 msec, and the mean conductance was 18 pS.

ACETYLCHOLINE RECEPTOR CHANNELS

One development that improved the quality of single-channel recordings was the observation that cells grown in tissue culture were better candidates for the patch-clamp technique than were natural tissues. This had to do with membrane infolding, which is seen in vivo, and connective tissue layers that frequently surround living cells. The earliest observations of single-channel currents in cultured vertebrate muscle cells appeared in *Nature* in 1979: Nelson and Sachs used the on-cell technique to record currents in avian skeletal muscle with a mean conductance of 60 pS and a mean open time around 10 msec at 22 °C. They also reported flickering, or opening and closing of channels during each "open" period, indicating a complex gating mechanism. Jackson and Lecar (1979) used a similar technique with cultured rat muscle fibers and observed single-channel currents such as those depicted in Figure 9. The mean conductance was 48 pS and the mean open time 3.2 msec, at 22 °C. Some flickering of open channels can be seen in the figure, as well as addition of currents from two channels open at the same time. Jackson and Lecar also showed that the distribution of open times was exponential, consistent with the idea that the closing of channels was a Poisson process (more in Chapter 12). Soon after this, Horn and Patlak (1980) applied the "inside-out"

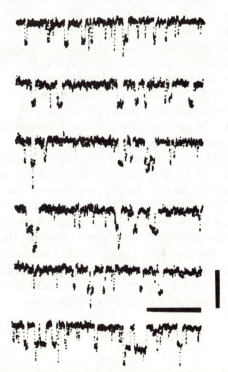

9

Single acetylcholine receptor channels in cultured rat muscle. On-cell recording technique, cell held at −90 mV with additional intracellular electrode. Patch pipette filled with 1 μM carbamylcholine. Scales 100 msec, 10 pA. (From Jackson and Lecar, 1979.)

method to record currents in an excised patch of cultured rat muscle. The mean channel conductance was 33.5 pS and open times were in the range of 2–10 msec.

One significant difference between the ACh channel and K^+ and Na^+ channels is the large permeability of the ACh channel to a wide variety of cations. Besides Na^+ and K^+, the channel admits Li^+, Cs^+, NH_4^+, Ca^{2+}, Sr^{2+}, Ba^{2+}, and Mg^{2+} (Adams et al., 1980). This is basically because the ACh receptor channel is larger in diameter than the Na^+ or K^+ channels. The structures of these ion-carrying channels will be compared in Chapter 13.

OTHER ION CHANNELS

By now, a great variety of channels has been studied with the various patch pipette techniques described above. Some of these are voltage-activated channels that are mainly permeable to calcium ions (Brown et al., 1982; Fenwick et al., 1982). Others are activated or inhibited by exposure to specific ligands such as glutamate (Patlak et al., 1979) or serotonin (Siegelbaum et al., 1982). In one ingenious application of the method, single pressure-sensitive channels have been studied in excised patches from cultured muscle cells (Guhary and Sachs, 1984). When the pressure in the pipette is increased or decreased, the membrane stretches or contracts and produces a burst of single-channel activity. These channels are not blocked by α-bungarotoxin, unlike the ACh receptor channels.

At this point we have not discussed the theory of gating of membrane ion channels. We have seen that different membranes have single channels that each admit about the same amount of current at a given potential. The rate of channel opening and closing increases with depolarization, and the large-scale currents in squid axons, muscle fibers, and other excitable cells can be explained by the summation of these miniature currents. Knowledge of this represents a considerable advance in our understanding of these systems, but the theories presented in the next chapter show how the channels are gated to produce the known behavior of intact, excitable cells.

PROBLEMS

1. Plot Equation 3 for $f = 10$ to 1000 Hz, if $c = 10^{-10}$ $V^2 \cdot sec$ and $f_c = 90$ Hz.
2. Now plot log $S'(f)$ versus log f for the data in Problem 1.
3. Add a component equal to $10^{-9}/f$ to the noise spectrum in Problem 2 and plot log $S(f)$ versus log f from 10 to 1000 Hz.

4. The current through a single Na^+ channel in a myoball membrane is given by $I = \gamma(E - E_{Na})$, where γ = single-channel conductance. If γ = 18 pS and E_{Na} = +100 mV, find I when E = -30 mV.

5. How many monovalent cations must cross the membrane per second to give this much current?

6. The mean channel open time in the myoball membrane is 0.7 msec. How many Na^+ ions cross the membrane during the average channel opening?

7. The peak inward current density in the above membrane is about 1 mA/cm^2. How many Na^+ channels per square micrometer must open at about the same time to give this current? (This is one estimate of the number of channels/μm^2.)

REFERENCES

Adams, D. J., Dwyer, T. M., and Hille, B. 1980. The permeability of endplate channels to monovalent and divalent metal cations. *J. Gen. Physiol.* 75, 493–510.

Anderson, C. R., and Stevens, C. F. 1973. Voltage clamp analysis of acetylcholine produced end–plate current fluctuations at frog neuromuscular junction. *J. Physiol.* 235, 655–691.

Barrett, J. N., Magleby, K. L., and Pallotta, B. S. 1982. Properties of single calcium-activated potassium channels in cultured rat muscle. *J. Physiol.* 331, 211–230.

Bean, R. C., Shepherd, W. C., Chan, H., and Eichner, J. T. 1969. Discrete conductance fluctuations in lipid bilayer protein membranes. *J. Gen. Physiol.* 53, 741–745.

Brown, A. M., Camerer, H., Kunze, D. L., and Lux, H. D. 1982. Similarity of unitary Ca^{2+} currents in three different species. *Nature (Lond.)* 299, 156–158.

Cooper, E., and Shrier, A. 1985. Single-channel analysis of fast transient potassium currents from rat nodose neurons. *J. Physiol.* 369, 199–208.

Conti, F., and Neher, E. 1980. Single channel recordings of K^+ currents in squid axons. *Nature (Lond.)* 285, 140–143.

DeFelice, L. J., and Michalides, J. P. L. M. 1972. Electrical noise from synthetic membranes. *J. Membr. Biol.* 9, 261–290.

Derksen, H. E., and Verveen, A. A. 1966. Fluctuations of resting neural membrane potential. *Science* 151, 1388–1389.

Ehrenstein, G., Lecar, H., and Nossal, R. 1970. The nature of the negative resistance in bimolecular lipid membranes containing excitability-inducing material. *J. Gen. Physiol.* 55, 119–133.

Eisenberg, M., Hall, J. E., and Mead, C. A. 1973. The nature of the voltage-dependent conductance induced by alamethicin in black lipid membranes. *J. Membr. Biol.* 14, 143–176.

Ewald, D., Williams, A., and Levitan, I. B. 1985. Modulation of single Ca^{++}-dependent K^+ channel activity by protein phosphorylation. *Nature (Lond.)* 315, 503–506.

Fenwick, E. M., Marty, A., and Neher, E. 1982. Sodium and calcium channels in bovine chromaffin cells. *J. Physiol.* 331, 599–635.

Fishman, H. M. 1973. Relaxation spectra of potassium channel noise from squid axon membranes. *Proc. Natl. Acad. Sci. USA* 70, 876–879.

Fishman, H. M., Moore, L. E., and Poussart, D. J. M. 1975. Potassium-ion conduction noise in squid axon membrane. *J. Membr. Biol.* 24, 305–328.

Guhary, F., and Sachs, F. 1984. Stretch-activated single ion channel currents in tissue-cultured embryonic chick skeletal muscle. *J. Physiol.* 352, 685–701.

Hamill, O. P., Marty, A., Neher, E., Sakmann, B., and Sigworth, F. J. 1981. Improved patch-clamp techniques for high-resolution current recording from cells and cell-free membrane patches. *Pflügers Arch. Gesamte Physiol. Menschen Tiere* 391, 85–100.

Hladky, S. B., and Haydon, D. A. 1970. Discreteness of conductance change in bimolecular lipid membranes in the presence of certain antibiotics. *Nature (Lond).* 225, 451–453.

Hooge, F. N., and Gaal, J. L. M. 1970. Fluctuations with a 1/f spectrum in the conductance of ionic solutions and in the voltage of concentration cells. *Phillips Res. Rep.* 26, 77–90.

Horn, R., and Patlak, J. 1980. Single channel currents from excised patches of muscle membrane. *Proc. Natl. Acad. Sci. USA* 77, 6930–6934.

Jackson, M. B., and Lecar, H. 1979. Single postsynaptic channel currents in tissue cultured muscle. *Nature (Lond.)* 282, 863–864.

Katz, B., and Miledi, R. 1971. Further observations on acetylcholine noise. *Nature New Biol.* 232, 124–126.

Katz, B., and Miledi, R. 1972. The statistical nature of the acetylcholine potential and its molecular components. *J. Physiol.* 224, 665–699.

Katz, B., and Miledi, R. 1973. The characteristics of "end-plate noise" produced by different depolarizing drugs. *J. Physiol.* 230, 707–717.

Mueller, P., and Rudin, D. O. 1963. Induced excitability in reconstituted cell membrane structure. *J. Theor. Biol.* 4, 268–280.

Mueller, P., and Rudin, D. O. 1968. Resting and action potentials in experimental bimolecular lipid membranes. *J. Theor. Biol.* 18, 222–258.

Neher, E., and Sakmann, B. 1976. Single-channel currents recorded from membrane of denervated frog muscle fibres. *Nature (Lond).* 260, 799–802.

Neher, E., and Stevens, C. F. 1977. Conductance fluctuations and ionic pores in membranes. *Ann. Rev. Biophys. Bioeng.* 6, 345–381.

Nelson, D. J., and Sachs, F. 1979. Single ionic channels observed in tissue-cultured muscle. *Nature (Lond).* 282, 861–863.

Patlak, J. B., Gration, K. A. F., and Usherwood, P. N. R. 1979. Single glutamate-activated channels in locust muscle. *Nature (Lond).* 278, 643–645.

Poussart, D. J. M. 1971 Membrane current noise in lobster axon under voltage clamp. *Biophys. J.* 11, 211–234.

Rice, S. O. 1944. Mathematical analysis of random noise. *Bell Syst. Tech. J.* 23, 282–332.

Sakmann, B., and Neher, E. 1983. *Single-Channel Recording.* New York, Plenum.

Siebenga, E., de Goede, J., and Verveen, A. A. 1974. The influence of TTX, DNP and TEA on membrane flicker noise and shot effect noise of the frog node of Ranvier. *Pflügers Arch. Gesamte Physiol. Menschen Tiere* 351, 25–34.

Siebenga, E., and Verveen, A. A. 1972. Membrane noise and ion transport in the node of Ranvier. *Biomembranes: Passive Permeability of Cell Membranes* (Vol. 3), F. Kreuzer and J. G. F. Slegers (eds.) New York, Plenum, 473–482.

Siegelbaum, S. A., Camardo, J. S., and Kandel, E. R. 1982. Serotonin and cyclic AMP close single K^+ channels in *Aplysia* sensory neurones. *Nature (Lond).* 299, 413–417.

Sigworth, F. J., and Neher, E. 1980. Single Na^+ channel currents observed in cultured rat muscle cells. *Nature (Lond.)* 287, 447–449.

Spangenberg, K. R. 1957. *Fundamentals of Electron Devices.* New York, McGraw-Hill.

Verveen, A. A. 1962. Axon diameter and fluctuations in excitability. *Acta Morphol. Neerl. Scand.* 5, 79–85.

Verveen, A. A., and Derksen, H. E. 1965. Fluctuations in membrane potential of axons and the problem of coding. *Kybernetik* 2, 152–160.

Verveen, A. A., Derksen, H. E., and Schick, K. L. 1967. Voltage fluctuations of neural membrane. *Nature (Lond).* 216, 588–589.

12

THEORIES OF SINGLE-CHANNEL
BEHAVIOR

The modern interpretation of single-channel currents as the building blocks of excitable-cell behaviors came about during the 1970s from three principal directions at almost the same time: (1) As mentioned in the last chapter, neurophysiologists were paying increased attention to the unitary events underlying electrical noise in nerve and muscle cells; (2) biophysicists were studying single-channel conductances in artificial membranes; and (3) intrepid researchers finally succeeded in recording these events in isolated patches of muscle membrane under controlled voltages. The progress in each of these areas will be discussed in a somewhat overlapping way, as the results themselves happened.

STATISTICS OF CHANNEL OPENING AND CLOSING

In a study of endplate noise, Stevens (1972) took a different approach from Katz and Miledi, who had assumed that the microscopic change in potential was exponential in form (see Chapter 11). Instead, Stevens used the model shown in Figure 1: Each channel is assumed to open at random and remain open for a random length of time. Each channel has only two conductance states: one where the conductance is zero and one where it is γ. It is assumed that there are N channels per unit area of membrane, each of which has an independent probability p of being open at any time. Then the number n of open channels is given by the binomial distribution. The average of n is

$$\bar{n} = Np \tag{1}$$

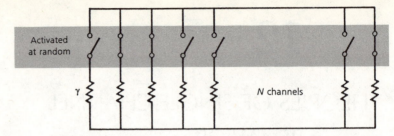

1

Random-switch model of membrane noise. Each channel adds an increment of γ to total membrane conductance. Switches indicate gates, activated at random. N channels/unit area of membrane.

The variance of the binomial distribution is

$$\sigma^2 = Np(1 - p) \tag{2}$$

Thus the mean total conductance is

$$\mu_g = Np\gamma \tag{3}$$

and the variance of the conductance is

$$\sigma_g^2 = \gamma^2\sigma^2 = \gamma^2Np(1 - p) \tag{4}$$

where σ_g is the standard deviation of the conductance.
Combining Equations 3 and 4 yields

$$\frac{\sigma_g^2}{\mu_g} = \gamma(1 - p) \tag{5}$$

For the condition where there is very low probability of a single channel opening, such as very low agonist concentration around the endplate receptors ($p << 1$), this becomes

$$\frac{\sigma_g^2}{\mu_g} = \gamma \tag{6}$$

Anderson and Stevens (1973) used this method to calculate the single-channel conductance of the muscle endplate channel under the action of ACh. The conductance statistics were obtained from voltage-clamp current measurements using the following relationships:

$$\mu_g = \frac{\mu_I}{V - V_{\text{eq}}} \tag{7}$$

$$\sigma_g^2 = \frac{\sigma_I^2}{(V - V_{eq})^2} \tag{8}$$

where μ_I = mean current
σ_I^2 = variance of current

The mean value of γ that they found for the ACh receptor channel in this way was 20.5 pS.

Begenisich and Stevens (1975) used essentially this approach to calculate the conductance of a single potassium channel in the node of Ranvier. The nerve fibers were treated with TTX to block sodium currents and subjected to depolarization under voltage clamp. If the channel is assumed to have only two conductance states (open or closed), the value of γ_K is 4 pS.

The conductance of a single sodium channel in the node was found by Sigworth (1977), using a clever extension of this method: He looked at changes in variance of currents in TEA- or cesium-treated nodes as a function of time after the start of a depolarizing step and plotted σ_I^2 versus μ_I. The data were interpreted with the random-switch model as follows: If there are N channels per unit area, each of which carries a current i at a certain membrane potential, the mean current is given by

$$\mu_I = Npi \tag{9}$$

where p is the probability that a channel is in its open state. The variance of the currents may be found by an argument parallel to that leading to Equation 4 as

$$\sigma_I^2 = Np(1 - p)i^2 \tag{10}$$

From Equations 9 and 10, the theoretical relationship of σ_I^2 and μ_I is

$$\sigma_I^2 = i\mu_I - \mu_I^2/N \tag{11}$$

From fits of Equation 11 to the observed curves of σ_I^2 versus μ_I, the single-channel conductance (equal to $i/[V - V_{eq}]$) was found to vary from 2.5 to 7.7 pS. The sodium and potassium channel conductances may also be found by a less direct method (discussed in the next sections).

ENDPLATE NOISE ANALYSIS

The spectral density functions for current fluctuations in voltage-clamped membranes may be calculated using a theorem of fluctuation analysis: The covariance function for the current $I(t)$ is defined as

$$C_I(\tau) = \lim_{T \to \infty} \frac{1}{T} \int_0^T [I(t) - \mu_I][I(t + \tau) - \mu_I]dt \tag{12}$$

where μ_I = mean current. (The autocorrelation function of a signal is equal to the covariance with the initial amplitude normalized to one.) By the WIENER-KHINCHIN THEOREM, the spectral density function for the fluctuations of current is related to the covariance function by

$$S_I(f) = \text{Re}\mathscr{F}[C_I(\tau)] \tag{13}$$

where Re$\mathscr{F}$ denotes the real part of the Fourier transform.

In practice, this is equal to

$$S_I(f) = 4 \int_0^\infty C_I(\tau) \cos(2\pi f \tau)d\tau \tag{14}$$

In other words, all of the information about the spectral density function (frequency domain) is contained in the covariance function (time domain). This property has been used instead of tuned filters to obtain the spectral density functions of noise signals. The covariance is computed digitally, and the spectrum obtained with a FAST FOURIER TRANSFORM routine used in engineering (Conti et al., 1975).

Anderson and Stevens (1973) used the kinetic model of Magleby and Stevens (1972) to interpret the acetylcholine-produced noise in the muscle endplate in terms of single-channel activity. The channels were assumed to open under the action of the transmitter as follows:

$$T + R \underset{}{\overset{K}{\rightleftharpoons}} T \cdot R \underset{\beta}{\overset{\alpha}{\rightleftharpoons}} T \cdot R^* \tag{15}$$

where T is the transmitter, ACh
R is the receptor
$T \cdot R$ is the complex associated with a closed channel
$T \cdot R^*$ is the complex associated with an open channel
α = rate constant for channel opening
β = rate constant for channel closing

Magleby and Stevens (1972) had shown that the time constant for decay of endplate currents was equal to $1/\beta$, where β was the rate constant for channel closing. Anderson and Stevens carried this further, showing that spontaneously occurring miniature endplate currents also decayed with this time constant and relating noise spectra produced by applied transmitter to the parameters of the model in Equation 15. The covariance function for the current noise was found as

$$C_I(\tau) = A e^{-\beta\tau} \qquad (16)$$

$$A = \mu_I \gamma (V - V_{eq})/N \qquad (17)$$

where μ_I = mean endplate current
γ = single-channel conductance
V = membrane potential
V_{eq} = reversal potential for the endplate current
N = number of channels per unit area

The covariance function for N channels is equal to $NC_I(\tau)$, so the spectral density function, from Equation 14, is

$$S_I(f) = 4NA \int_0^\infty e^{-\beta\tau}\cos(2\pi f\tau)d\tau \qquad (18)$$

Integrating directly,

$$S_I(f) = \frac{2NA/\beta}{1 + (2\pi f/\beta)^2} \qquad (19)$$

Substituting for A,

$$S_I(f) = \frac{2\mu_I\gamma(V - V_{eq})/\beta}{1 + (2\pi f/\beta)^2} \qquad (20)$$

which has the same form as that observed experimentally (Figure 3, Chapter 11).

The useful features of this expression are the zero-frequency value $S_I(0)$, and the corner frequency $\beta/2\pi$. When $f = 0$,

$$S_I(0) = 2\mu_I\gamma(V - V_{eq})/\beta \qquad (21)$$

from which γ may be found as

$$\gamma = \frac{S_I(0)\beta}{2\mu_I(V - V_{eq})} \qquad (22)$$

The value of γ found by Anderson and Stevens using this method was 32 pS, or somewhat larger than that obtained with Equation 6. They regarded the higher value as a better estimate since it was obtained under better voltage-clamp conditions. The corner frequency, f_c, is that for which $S_I(f) = S_I(0)/2$. It provides a means of measuring β, the rate constant for channel closing, which is also the inverse of the mean channel open time. Thus,

$$\beta = 2\pi f_c \tag{23}$$

Furthermore, by measuring f_c at different membrane potentials, it was found that β varied with potential according to

$$\beta = Be^{AV} \tag{24}$$

where A and B are constants. This is precisely the relationship found by Magleby and Stevens (1972) for the closing rate constant in their study of muscle endplate currents.

In a similar study, Neher and Sakmann (1975) showed that the relaxation time constant for endplate currents in the presence of cholinergic drugs was the same as that obtained from drug-induced fluctuations. Both this and the above studies of noise spectra provided important confirmations of the single-channel theory of endplate conductance.

SINGLE-CHANNEL CURRENTS IN ARTIFICIAL MEMBRANES

A much stronger confirmation that ionic channels could be described by models with quantized conductances came from the first direct measurements of single-channel currents, in artificial membranes. After Ehrenstein et al. (1970) demonstrated single-channel currents in bilayers treated with the proteinaceous extract excitability inducing material (EIM), they developed the following model of gating of these channels:

$$C \underset{\beta}{\overset{\alpha}{\rightleftharpoons}} O \tag{25}$$

where C = closed state
O = open state
α = rate constant for channel opening
β = rate constant for channel closing

The rate of change of probability of a channel being in the open state is given by (Jackson et al., 1983)

$$dp_O/dt = \alpha p_C - \beta p_O \tag{26}$$

where $p_C + p_O = 1$. (This is basically the same as the Hodgkin-Huxley equations for ionic currents; see Equations 3, 6, and 7, Chapter 6.) The solution is

$$p_O = K\,e^{-t/\tau} + \alpha\tau \tag{27}$$

where K = a constant
   $\tau = 1/(\alpha + \beta)$

The constant K is adjusted to fit the initial conditions, i.e., whether the probability is starting at zero at time $t = $ o (activation) or at some finite value and then decreasing (relaxation).

If·we assume that the rate constants change instantaneously with changes in potential, then the conductance relaxes according to

$$g = N\gamma(K\ e^{-t/\tau} + \alpha\tau) \tag{28}$$

where N = number of channels per unit area
   γ = single-channel conductance

In other words, for the model in Equation 25, the relaxation time constant is equal to the inverse of the sum of the rate constants. In the usual experimental conditions, the relaxation of current is studied upon changing to a new potential where α is much smaller than β; then the relaxation time constant is given by

$$\tau \approx 1/\beta \tag{29}$$

Besides describing the current relaxations, this model also predicts the distribution of channel open-times, that is, the length of time single channels stay open once they have opened (Ehrenstein et al., 1974). This may be derived as follows: The probability of an open channel closing in a very short time dt is βdt, where β is the rate constant for channel closing. If this probability is homogeneous (roughly constant) over time, and the parameters that determine it (and β) do not change with time so that the probability of closing is independent of past history of the system, then the closing behaves like a POISSON PROCESS (Feller, 1968). One can define $P(t)$ as the probability of an open channel staying open longer than time t. Then the probability of staying open longer than $t + dt$ is

$$P(t + dt) = P(t)(1 - \beta dt) \tag{30}$$

where $1 - \beta dt$ = probability of not closing in dt.

Rearranging,

$$\frac{P(t + dt) - P(t)}{dt} = -\beta P(t) \tag{31}$$

As $dt \to 0$, this becomes

$$\frac{dP(t)}{dt} = -\beta P(t) \tag{32}$$

The solution of this is

$$P(t) = e^{-\beta t} \tag{33}$$

This is the cumulative distribution function for a Poisson process. The probability density function is given by the derivative

$$P'(t) = \beta e^{-\beta t} \tag{34}$$

This is the probability density function for an opening lasting between t and $t + dt$. The average open time, t_o, is found as

$$t_o = \int_0^\infty \beta t e^{-\beta t} dt = 1/\beta \tag{35}$$

This result equates the mean channel open time with the time constant for relaxation of macroscopic currents (Equation 29). It is a fundamental step in relating the membrane electrical properties to the opening and closing of membrane ionic channels and has been used to analyze single-channel data in many nerve and muscle preparations (Dionne and Leibowitz, 1982; Quandt and Narahashi, 1982; Jackson, 1986).

DELAYED RECTIFIER POTASSIUM CHANNELS

Equation 25 for the EIM channel is basically a two-state (open-close) model. This type of scheme was insufficient to account for delayed (potassium) currents in a structure such as the squid axon, which turn on more slowly (with higher-order kinetics). To analyze the fluctuations seen in K^+ currents of the squid axon, Hill and Chen (1972) used a model with two closed states leading to an open state:

$$C_1 \underset{\beta}{\overset{2\alpha}{\rightleftharpoons}} C_2 \underset{2\beta}{\overset{\alpha}{\rightleftharpoons}} O \tag{36}$$

The equations governing the transitions from a given state are

$$dp_{C_1}/dt = \beta p_{C_2} - 2\alpha p_{C_1} \tag{37}$$

$$dp_{C_2}/dt = 2\alpha p_{C_1} - \beta p_{C_2} + 2\beta p_O - \alpha p_{C_2} \tag{38}$$

$$dp_O/dt = \alpha p_{C_2} - 2\beta p_o \tag{39}$$

where C_1 is the first closed state
C_2 is the second closed state
O is the open state
α and β are rate constants for opening and closing

The solution for the probability of channels being in the open state, starting from being closed, is

$$p_O = (\alpha\tau)^2(1 - e^{-t/\tau})^2 \tag{40}$$

where $\tau = 1/(\alpha + \beta)$.

The membrane conductance is given by

$$g_K = N\gamma p_O \tag{41}$$

where N = number of channels per unit area
γ = single-channel conductance

This is quite similar to the Hodgkin-Huxley potassium conductance (Equations 2 and 4, Chapter 6), only the argument is raised to the second power. The model in Equation 36 is an energetic representation of some physical process that is as yet unknown. The transition from the first closed state to the second might consist, for instance, of a discrete conformational change of the channel that does not open the pore sufficiently to admit K^+ ions. The time required for some channels to enter this state before entering the open state would explain the slow rise of the outward current.

Using this model, the spectral density function of the noise was calculated and compared with that from real axons. These authors concluded that $1/f$ noise in the squid axon was mainly due to current through *open* K^+ channels, and not the open-close kinetics of the channels.

SODIUM CHANNELS

The sodium-carrying mechanism has an additional feature to that found in the delayed rectifier channels, namely, the current inactivates with a maintained step of potential. A simple model that can explain this behavior is

$$C \underset{\beta_1}{\overset{\alpha_1}{\rightleftharpoons}} O \underset{k_2}{\overset{k_1}{\rightleftharpoons}} I \tag{42}$$

where C is the resting closed state
O is the open state
I is a closed (inactivated) state
α_1, β_1, k_1, and k_2 are rate constants

The activation process occurs by starting out with most of the channels in the C state, which is determined by the values of the rate constants at the holding potential. When the potential is stepped to the test value, the rate constants change instantaneously, and the average occupancy (probability of being in a given state) shifts from state C to O, and finally to I. Only state O is conducting, so the sodium conductance is given by

$$g_{Na} = N\gamma p_O \tag{43}$$

where N = number of channels per unit area
  γ = single-channel conductance
  p_O = probability of being in the open state

The physical realization of the inactivation process is also obscure but may involve either a blockage or change in size of the channel pore when it is in the I-state.

  This simple model does not account for the slow initial rise of the sodium conductance, described by the m^3 dependence in the Hodgkin-Huxley theory (Equation 5, Chapter 6). From their studies of single Na^+ channels in cultured pituitary cells (Horn et al. 1984), Horn and Vandenberg (1984) chose the following kinetic model as best describing the behavior of these channels:

$$
\begin{array}{c}
I \\
\diagup \quad \diagdown \\
C_1 \rightleftharpoons C_2 \rightleftharpoons C_3 \rightleftharpoons O
\end{array}
\tag{44}
$$

where C_1, C_2, and C_3 are closed states of the channel
  O is a single open state
  I is an inactivated state

They found no evidence for more than one open state, based on amplitude histograms of single-channel currents. After comparing the statistical properties of 25 different models, they decided the one above best described the open- and closed-time distributions, and the inactivation properties of the macroscopic (whole cell) currents. The solution for this model is somewhat cumbersome to derive, and it is easier to write the differential equations for each state, in the same way as Equations 37–39, and solve them numerically on a computer.

ACETYLCHOLINE RECEPTOR CHANNELS

A complicating factor in applying this theory to the acetylcholine receptor is that the associated channels apparently open in bursts of varying length (Colquhoun and Sakmann, 1983; Auerbach and Sachs, 1983; Sine and Steinbach, 1984). To explain this behavior, more complicated models have been put forth, involving more than one closed state. Colquhoun and Sakmann (1983) used a model similar to that of Anderson and Stevens (1973) (Equation 15, above), but assuming *two* closed states of the receptor:

$$R \rightleftharpoons TR \xrightarrow[k_{-2}]{k_{+2}} T_2R \xrightarrow[\beta]{\alpha} T_2R^* \qquad (45)$$

where R is the receptor
T is the transmitter
TR is the complex with one transmitter molecule (closed)
T_2R is the complex with two transmitters (closed)
T_2R^* is the complex with the channel open
α = rate constant for channel opening
β = rate constant for channel closing

This model allows for bursts by saying that an open channel may close and then reopen, jumping between the T_2R and T_2R^* states. It also accounts for the agonist concentration dependence of the endplate conductance. Since the conductance increases approximately with the square of the transmitter concentration (Adams, 1975; Dionne et al., 1978), apparently two agonist molecules must bind to each receptor to cause it to open. Models similar to Equation 45 have been used by other authors (Dionne and Liebowitz, 1982; Hille, 1992; Horn, 1984) to explain the burst pattern of opening seen in the ACh receptor.

BLOCKAGE BY LOCAL ANESTHETICS

As mentioned in Chapter 7, one of the ways in which local anesthetics block conduction and excitation in nerve is by greatly reducing the inward sodium currents and attenuating the action potential. The first demonstration of the effect of local anesthetics on single-channel currents was that of Neher and Steinbach (1978), using denervated frog muscle. This is shown in Figure 2. Trace A shows currents recorded in the presence of suberyldicholine, an acetylcholine-like drug. In trace B the local anesthetic QX-222 was added, and the concentration was increased in traces C and D. The result was that the anesthetic disrupted the single-channel currents into bursts of much shorter, and therefore less effective, pulses. This behavior is called "flickering" and is presumably due to blocking of open endplate channels by the anesthetics.

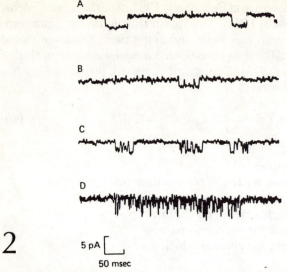

Effect of local anesthetic on single-channel current in chronically denervated muscle. Suberyldicholine applied in all traces. Anesthetic (QX-222) concentration 0 in A, 5 μM in B, 10 μM in C, and 50 μM in D. (From Neher and Steinbach, 1978.)

The kinetic scheme generally used to explain block by local anesthetics is a modification of Equation 45:

$$R \rightleftharpoons TR \rightleftharpoons T_2R \rightleftharpoons T_2R^* \rightleftharpoons QXT_2R^* \qquad (46)$$

where QXT_2R^* is a blocked state. The channel flickers between the open state T_2R^* and the blocked state as the anesthetic enters and leaves the channel.

MODIFICATIONS OF THEORIES FROM SINGLE-CHANNEL OBSERVATIONS

One of the dramatic results of patch-clamp studies has been the direct observation of channel properties that affect macroscopic currents in whole cells. Some parts of the theories of activation and inactivation that previously had to be taken as assumptions could now be tested directly. Among these was the idea, implicit in the Hodgkin-Huxley theory, that activation and inactivation were separate processes. As mentioned in Chapter 7, these workers had assumed no coupling at all between the activation variable m and the inactivation variable h.

However, others had proposed tightly coupled activation and inactivation processes in which channels had to go through an active state before becoming inactivated (Moore and Jakobsson, 1971; Bezanilla and Armstrong, 1977). The recording of single-channel Na^+ currents in patches from cultured muscle cells (Horn et al., 1981) gave strong evidence as to which interpretation was correct.

These investigators first applied 144 depolarizations to the patch, and calculated the probability $P(t)$ that a sodium channel was open t seconds after the beginning of a depolarizing pulse. This function resembled the macroscopic sodium current in shape, i.e., peaked about 1 msec after the start of the depolarization and then decreased to zero. They then plotted the conditional probability $P(T,t)$ of a channel being open t seconds after the last opening, where T was the time since the start of the depolarization before any opening occurred. If the inactivation occurred only after an opening, then the conditional probability should have been the same as $P(t)$ but shifted to the right by T. Their result, however, showed that the conditional probability of a channel being open T seconds after the depolarization was the same whether or not the channels had opened during that time. The inactivation process had taken place as a result of depolarization, not of opening; Hodgkin and Huxley were right.

Another question that can be answered from patch-clamp studies is: When sodium inactivation is removed by treatment with agents like pronase (Chapter 7), what happens to the individual Na^+ channels? Does the distribution of open and closed times change or is the single-channel conductance increased? One result is shown in Figure 3, taken from sodium channels in inside-out patches from myotubes (Patlak and Horn, 1982). The top trace in the control records is the membrane potential; below it, three current records are shown in response to repetitions of the depolarizing pulse. The average channel open time was 3.2 msec. When N-bromoacetamide (NBA) was added to the "internal" solution around the patch, the records in the bottom part were obtained. As seen in these bottom three current records, the mean channel open time was greatly increased (to a value of 29 msec) by this agent, which also removed the inactivation from the macroscopic records. The channel conductance was not affected by NBA. Almost the same results were obtained when the patches were treated with pronase. Thus, removal of inactivation by treatment with these chemicals was a result of a large prolongation of the time that sodium channels spent in the open state. These findings were consistent with a kinetic model in which the rate constant leading back from the open state to the last closed state was slower than that expected from the Hodgkin-Huxley model.

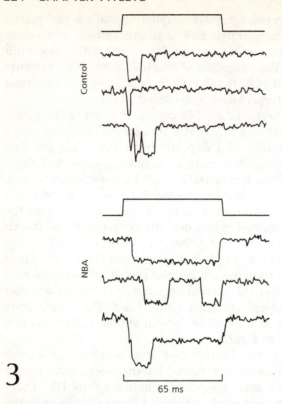

3

65 ms

Effect of *N*-bromoacetamide (NBA) on sodium channel currents in excised patches from rat myotubes. Outward currents blocked with cesium ions in "external" solution; NBA removes Na$^+$ inactivation (sag) in whole-membrane currents. Top traces are potential, stepped from −110 mV to +50 mV. Next traces are currents produced by three repetitions of voltage step. (Amplitude of potential pulse also indicates current scale of 1 pA.) "Control": Single Na$^+$ channel currents. "NBA": large increase in channel open time produced by treatment with 300μ*M* NBA. (From Patlak and Horn, 1982).

Thus, after several years of model-making to explain currents in whole cells and artificial membranes, and the fluctuations that were later seen in those currents, it has become possible to measure the unitary events directly. What was once only speculation—the timing of opening and closing of single channels, for instance—is now observable. It is important to note that, while we can measure channel currents, our ideas of how channel molecules behave are still based on theoretical models. Progress to date has depended both on technical improvements, such as the patch clamp, and theoretical advances to interpret the single-channel data. In the next chapter, we shall go one step further and examine some recent findings about the molecular structure of ion channels and how these structures are genetically determined.

PROBLEMS

1. With a certain concentration of applied acetylcholine, the mean and standard deviation of conductance in the frog motor endplate are 3×10^{-6} S and 8.4×10^{-9} S^2. Find the single-channel conductance.

2. In Anderson and Stevens's model (Equation 22), the parameters appropriate to a real endplate are $S_I(0) = 2.33 \times 10^{-21}$ $A^2 \cdot$sec, $f_c = 21$ Hz, $\mu_I = -80$ nA, $V = -60$ mV, and $V_{eq} = 0$. What is the single-channel conductance?

3. In the model of an EIM channel in Equation 25, if $\alpha = 1.0$/sec and $\beta = 25$/sec, what is the time constant for relaxation of macroscopic currents?

4. What is the mean channel open time from probabilistic arguments (Equation 35)?

5. The probabilities of a potassium channel being in each state in the model of Equation 36 are p_{C1}, p_{C2}, and p_O. What mathematical relation must always be true for these state probabilities?

6. Suppose the channel in Problem 5 is held at a depolarized potential where β is very small compared to α. What state will eventually have the greatest probability of occupation?

7. Write the general expression for the macroscopic potassium current I_K in terms of the peak conductance $\bar{g}_K$, the membrane potential E, the potassium equilibrium potential E_K, and one of the probabilities in Problem 5.

REFERENCES

Adams, P. 1975. An analysis of the dose-response curve at voltage clamped frog endplates. *Pflügers Arch. Gesamte Physiol. Menschen Tiere* 360, 145–153.

Anderson, C. R. and Stevens, C. F. 1973. Voltage clamp analysis of acetylcholine produced end-plate current fluctuations at frog neuromuscular junction. *J. Physiol.* 235, 655–691.

Auerbach, A. and Sachs, F. 1983. Flickering of a nicotinic ion channel to a subconductance state. *Biophys. J.* 42, 1–10.

Begenisich, T. and Stevens, C. F. 1975. How many conductance states do potassium channels have? *Biophys. J.* 15, 843–846.

Bezanilla, F. and Armstrong, C. M. 1977. Inactivation of the sodium channel I. Sodium current experiments. *J. Gen. Physiol.* 70, 549–566.

Colquhoun, D. and Sakmann, B. 1983. Bursts of openings in transmitter-activated ion channels. *Single-Channel Recording.* B. Sakmann and E. Neher (eds.). New York, Plenum, 345–364.

Conti, F., DeFelice, L. J. and Wanke, E. 1975. Potassium and sodium ion current noise in the membrane of the squid giant axon. *J. Physiol.* 248, 45–82.

Dionne, V. E. and Leibowitz, M. D. 1982. Acetylcholine receptor kinetics: a description from single-channel currents at snake neuromuscular junctions. *Biophys. J.* 39, 253–261.

Dionne, V. E., Steinbach, J. H. and Stevens, C. F. 1978. An analysis of the dose-response relationship at voltage-clamped frog neuromuscular junctions. *J. Physiol.* 281, 421–444.

Ehrenstein, G., Lecar, H. and Nossal, R. 1970. The nature of the negative resistance in bimolecular lipid membranes containing excitability-inducing material. *J. Gen. Physiol.* 55, 119–133.

Ehrenstein, G., Blumenthal, R., Latorre, R. and Lecar, H. 1974. Kinetics of the opening and closing of individual excitability-inducing material channels in a lipid bilayer. *J. Gen. Physiol.* 63, 707–721.

Feller, W. 1968. *An Introduction to Probability Theory and Its Applications*, 2nd ed., v. I. New York, Wiley.

Hill, T. L. and Chen, Y.-D. 1972. On the theory of ion transport across the nerve membrane IV. Noise from the open-close kinetics of K^+ channels. *Biophys. J.* 12, 948–959.

Hille, B. 1992. *Ionic Channels of Excitable Membranes*, Second Edition. Sunderland, Mass., Sinauer.

Horn, R. 1984. Gating of channels in nerve and muscle: a stochastic approach. *Ion Channels: Molecular and Physiological Aspects*. W. D. Stein (ed.). Orlando, Fla., Academic, 53–97.

Horn, R., Patlak, J. and Stevens, C. F. 1981. Sodium channels need not open before they inactivate. *Nature (Lond.)* 291, 426–427.

Horn, R. and Vandenberg, C. A. 1984. Statistical properties of single sodium channels. *J. Gen. Physiol.* 84, 505–534.

Horn, R., Vandenberg, C. A. and Lange, K. 1984. Statistical analysis of single sodium channels. Effects of *N*-bromoacetamide. *Biophys. J.* 45, 323–335.

Jackson, M. B. 1986. Toward a mechanism of gating of chemically activated channels. *Basic Mechanisms of the Epilepsies: Molecular and Cellular Approaches*. A. V. Delgado-Escueta, A. A. Ward, D. M. Woodbury and R. J. Porter (eds.). New York, Raven, 171–198.

Jackson, M. B., Lecar, H., Morris, C. E. and Wong, B. S. 1983. Single-channel current recording in excitable cells. *Current Methods in Cellular Neurobiology, v. III: Electrophysiological and Optical Recording Techniques*. J. L. Barker and J. F. McKelvy (eds.). New York, Wiley, 61–99.

Magleby, K. L. and Stevens, C. F. 1972. A quantitative description of end-plate currents. *J. Physiol.* 223, 173–197.

Moore, L. E. and Jakobsson, E. 1971. Interpretation of the sodium permeability changes of myelinated nerve in terms of linear relaxation theory. *J. Theor. Biol.* 33, 77–89.

Neher, E. and Sakmann, B. 1975. Voltage-dependence of drug-induced conductance in frog neuromuscular junction. *Proc. Natl. Acad. Sci. USA* 72, 2140–2144.

Neher, E. and Steinbach, J. H. 1978. Local anesthetics transiently block currents through single acetylcholine-receptor channels. *J. Physiol.* 277, 153–176.

Patlak, J. and Horn, R. 1982. Effect of N-bromoacetamide on single sodium channel currents in excised membrane patches. *J. Gen. Physiol.* 79, 333–351.

Quandt, F. N. and Narahashi, T. 1982. Modification of single Na^+ channels by batrachotoxin. *Proc. Natl. Acad. Sci. USA* 79, 6732–6736.

Sigworth, F. 1977. Sodium channels in nerve apparently have two conductance states. *Nature (Lond.)* 270, 265–267.

Sine, S. M. and Steinbach, J. H. 1984. Activation of nicotinic acetylcholine receptor. *Biophys. J.* 45, 175–185.

Stevens, C. F. 1972. Inferences about membrane properties from electrical noise measurements. *Biophys. J.* 12, 1028–1047.

13

STRUCTURAL BASIS OF CHANNEL
FUNCTION

Since we are now aware that physiologically important currents are carried by packets of ions flowing through open membrane channels, the next step in understanding channel behavior is a detailed knowledge of the atomic and molecular structures involved. Some of the questions we may ask about the channels include (1) how many there are per unit area, (2) how large they are, (3) what the single-channel conductance is, and (4) what structural features account for selectivity, gating, and blocking by anesthetics and other agents. Many of these questions were asked in the early stages of electrical recording from single neurons and muscle cells, and some important inferential results came from these studies (Hille, 1970). Recently, however, the identification of DNA sequences associated with specific channel proteins has led to much more sophisticated analysis of channel structures. (Fortunately, the electrophysiological results were available to confirm or refute the suggestions of these molecular studies.) In the first part of this chapter we shall recapitulate some of the results from electrophysiology that bear on channel structure and behavior.

DENSITY OF CHANNELS

As mentioned in Chapter 7, the process of ionic current conduction may be broken down into a *gating* mechanism, which allows ions to flow down their concentration gradients across membranes, and a *selectivity filter*, which discriminates between the various cations and anions for particular functions. The idea of gating was discussed by Hodgkin and Huxley as early as 1952. Some sort of charged particle or molecule had to reside in the membrane, to "sense" changes in the membrane potential, or field strength, and regulate the ionic currents. Hodgkin and Huxley (1952) calculated that a total of six electronic charges must cross the membrane for sodium ions to cross. (These could be individual charged particles or charges on a larger molecular structure.) Subsequently, the minuscule currents produced by the movement of these gating charges were measured (Armstrong and Bezanilla, 1973), confirming their existence. The DENSITY OF CHANNEL GATES in the membrane was estimated by dividing the integral of the gating charge during a voltage-clamp step by the electronic charge times the assumed value of six gating charges per channel (Chapter 7). The SINGLE-CHANNEL CONDUCTANCE was then estimated by dividing the typical macroscopic conductance by this channel density. Confirmations of the ballpark values of single-channel conductances also came from studies with binding of channel-blocking agents (Chapter 7) and membrane noise (Chapter 12).

CHANNEL SIZE

The size of the channel opening, or "pore", was then estimated from studies with ion selectivity (Hille, 1975a). This at first posed a paradox: If one examined the radii of all of the organic and inorganic cations that could pass through the sodium channel, the minimum pore size was about 3×5 Å (Hille, 1971, 1972). Na^+ ions apparently crossed the pore in partial association with some water molecules, and the channel was much more permeable to Na^+ ions than to K^+ ions. The potassium channel was smaller, perhaps a circle of diameter between 2.96 and 3.38 Å (Hille, 1973), and it passed K^+ ions but excluded Na^+. Yet the unhydrated radius of the sodium ion was smaller than that of the potassium ion (0.98 Å compared to 1.33 Å; Chapter 3). In later interpretations, the K^+ ion is considered to traverse K^+ channels in an almost unhydrated state, while the Na^+ ion is accompanied by at least one water molecule in the Na^+ channel (Hille, 1975a). The interaction of ions in solution with pores in membranes is more complex than the image of particles falling through a hole. (Although, in the acetylcholine receptor channel, which has an apparent dimension of 6.5×6.5 Å, almost no selectivity is seen among cations [Dwyer et al., 1980].)

GATING SITES

The discovery that internal application of the proteolytic enzymes called pronase could remove Na^+ inactivation in the squid axon (Chapter 7) strongly suggested that the inactivation (or h) gate was located on the axoplasmic side of the membrane. Eaton et al. (1978) carried this approach one step further, showing that arginine-specific reagents applied to the inside of the squid axon removed Na^+ inactivation. This result indicated that arginine residues in a peptide chain could in fact serve as the inactivation gates.

LOCATION OF BLOCKING SITES

From experiments with LOCAL ANESTHETIC BLOCK of K^+ channels, Armstrong and Hille (1972) concluded that the blocking site was within the pore, accessible to drug molecules in the axoplasm only when the channel was open (Chapter 7). This fairly detailed structural interpretation came from the observation that local anesthetics blocked almost exclusively from inside the cell membranes and showed USE-DEPENDENT BLOCK (Chapter 7).

Strichartz (1973) adapted the Woodhull (1973) model of channel blocking by protons to explain the voltage-sensitive behavior of Na^+ channel inhibition by quaternary ammonium compounds: The complexing of local anesthetic, QX, to open channels, C_o, is assumed to be the voltage-dependent step:

$$C_o + QX \overset{E}{\rightleftharpoons} C_o \cdot QX \tag{1}$$

where $C_o \cdot QX$ = blocked channels
E = membrane potential

The association constant for the blocking reaction, K_a, is

$$K_a = \frac{[C_o \cdot QX]}{[C_o][QX]} = K_0 e^{zF\delta E/RT} \tag{2}$$

where E = membrane potential
K_o = dissociation constant when $E = 0$
z = charge on the anesthetic ion
F = Faraday constant
δ = fraction of the applied potential E that affects the reaction

It is assumed that the electric field (voltage drop/distance) is constant in the membrane, so the factor δ is interpreted as the fraction of the membrane width at which the blocking site is located in the channel. Since RT/F is about 24 mV at the temperature at which these experiments were done (6°C) and the charge on the local anesthetic molecule is +1, Equation 2 reduces to

$$\frac{[C_o \cdot QX]}{[C_o][QX]} = K_0 e^{\delta E/24} \tag{3}$$

The sum of the numbers of blocked and unblocked channels is always equal to $[C_{total}]$, the total number of channels:

$$[C_o] + [C_o \cdot QX] = [C]_{total} \tag{4}$$

From Equations 3 and 4, the number of unblocked channels may be found as

$$[C_o] = \frac{[C]_{total}}{1 + K_o[QX]e^{\delta E/24}} \tag{5}$$

If the potential is held at two different conditioning potentials, E_1 and E_2, and then depolarized to a test potential E_t, the ratio of the peak Na^+ currents at E_t is

$$\frac{I(E_1)}{I(E_2)} = \frac{1 + K_o[QX]e^{\delta E_2/24}}{1 + K_o[QX]e^{\delta E_1/24}} \tag{6}$$

From fits of this relationship to peak Na^+ currents at different conditioning potentials, Strichartz concluded that the local anesthetic binding site was located about halfway between the inside and the outside of the channel.

INFERENCES ABOUT CHANNEL STRUCTURE

To explain the known properties of active sodium channels in the node of Ranvier, Hille (1975b) used a four-barrier Eyring-type model, shown in Figure 1. The channel itself is diagrammed on the right side of the

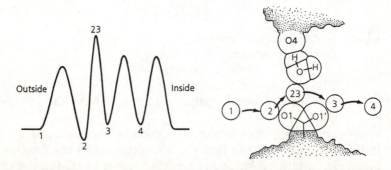

Molecular model of sodium channel in node of Ranvier. Left: Eyring model showing energy barriers encountered by Na^+ ion approaching the channel. Right: atoms drawn to scale of corresponding crystal radii. Oxygens O1 and O1' in carboxyl group. A water molecule is temporarily bonded to the O4 atom. See text for details. (From Hille, 1975b.)

figure. A carboxyl group sits on one side, with two oxygen atoms pointing toward the channel lumen. An oxygen group on the other side is able to interact with water molecules as they detach from the cations passing by. (It is likely that the interior negative charges of such channels are oxygens, since these are abundant and attract ions non-covalently.)

The energy barriers on the left side explain the electrostatic forces encountered by the traversing ions: The hydrated ion in water, surrounded by one or more shells of water molecules, is state 1. As the ion approaches the first oxygen atom in the —COO$^-$ group, it loses some water molecules but is stabilized by its attraction to the O1 atom; this is the bound state 2. Next the ion enters the narrow part of the channel, the selectivity filter. More water molecules are lost and a high-energy complex 23 is formed. The selectivity for Na$^+$ over K$^+$ arises from the difference in closeness of approach of the ions to the O atom (similar to the Eisenman selectivity theory discussed in Chapter 3). The ion then passes through the filter and acquires some more water molecules, forming state 3. More water is acquired (state 4), and, finally, the last, or axoplasmic, state is reached. This model, in its molecular detail, was formed completely from electrophysiological results, and from a guided intuition of what "must be."

ACETYLCHOLINE RECEPTORS

We have seen how ion channel structures were deduced from studies such as those above. The next step was to apply biochemical techniques to extracts of fractionated excitable membranes and try to isolate the channels themselves. This was first accomplished with the acetylcholine receptor (or AChR). Using the fact that radioactively labeled α-bungarotoxin binds covalently (irreversibly) to ACh receptors, Karlsson et al. (1972) and Raftery (1973) attached toxin molecules to a sepharose column and extracted the AChR from detergent-treated fragments of *Torpedo* electroplax. The receptor molecules contained four different polypeptide subunits, called α, β, γ, and δ, with molecular weights of 40, 50, 60, and 65 kDa. The structure was a pentamer with stoichiometry α$_2$βγδ (Raftery et al., 1980).

In order to be sure these protein fractions were actually acetylcholine receptors, Lindstrom et al. (1980) and Wu et al. (1981) prepared reconstituted lipid vesicles that contained the AChR in the membranes. These studies showed that ion fluxes across the receptors were stimulated by application of the ACh agonist, carbamylcholine.

In another approach to structure of the AChR, Ross et al. (1977) made pellets of receptor-rich membrane and did x-ray scattering experiments on them. One result was that the receptor protein extended asymmetrically across the membrane, protruding 55 Å on one side and 15 Å on the other. The overall length normal to the membrane was 110 Å. A repeat unit of 5.2 Å in the structure indicated the presence of α helices. From enhanced images of uranyl-stained pellets, they also showed that the receptors had a "rosette" form with subunits apparently arranged around a central pore. Then Klymkowsky and Stroud (1979) used a negative-staining technique of electron microscopy to visualize the receptors from the side, at the edge of a folded-over membrane vesicle. The funnel-shaped structures that they saw protruded about 50 Å on the outside of the membrane, in agreement with the predictions of Ross et al., above.

From computer-filtered images of uranyl-stained AChR membrane sheets, Kistler et al. (1982) produced the image of a typical ACh receptor channel shown in Figure 2. Part A shows the amount of protrusion of the receptor mouth on the external side of the membrane, and the presumed arrangement of the five subunits is shown in Part B. This structure was obtained from computer processing of electron microscope images, independent of results from electrophysiology.

GENOTYPE OF THE ACETYLCHOLINE RECEPTOR

The next big step in analyzing the structure of the acetylcholine receptor was sequencing the genes responsible for synthesis of the subunits. Noda et al. (1982) prepared complementary DNA from electroplax messenger RNA and obtained the base sequence of the gene. From this they deduced the amino acid structure of the α subunit. It consisted of 461 amino acids, and the predicted molecular weight was 50,116 Da. By plotting the hydrophilicity profile of the amino acids vs. position in the molecule, Noda et al. obtained the graph shown in Figure 3. The hydrophobic regions (value < 0) reside in the membrane, and the boxes below are secondary structures, some of which span the membrane.

In a subsequent study, Noda et al. (1983a, 1983b) elucidated the structures of the β, δ, and γ subunits, and found a large degree of homology between the four types of subunits. From examination of the hydrophilicity profiles, they concluded that each type of subunit contained four membrane-spanning segments (M1–M4) that could be part of the ion channel, as shown in Figure 4. The polypeptide molecule that forms each subunit wanders back and forth across the cell membrane, so that the hydrophilic regions are on the inside and outside, and the hydrophobic regions are in the membrane. Similar structures were proposed for the β, γ, and δ subunits. The subunits are arranged

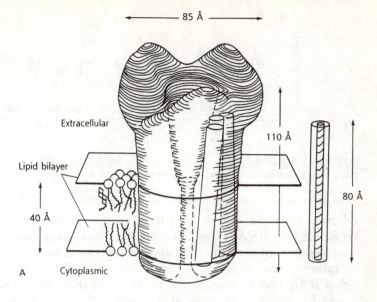

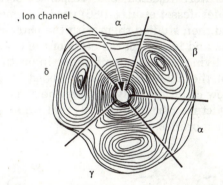

2

Three-dimensional model of acetylcholine receptor channel, based on computer filtered images of tubular lattices formed from suspensions of receptors. (From Kistler et al., 1982.)

linearly in the drawing, but it is suggested that they are actually in close apposition in the membrane and form the membrane AChR channel. We are thus provided with basic evidence about receptor-channel structure.

An even more dramatic confirmation that the cDNA that was cloned corresponded to the ACh receptor was provided by the work of Mishina et al. (1984). They prepared four mRNAs for the different

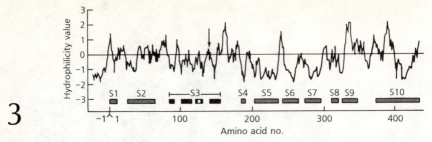

3

Hydrophilicity profile of α-subunit of ACh receptor. Membrane-spanning regions are those with values < 0. (From Noda et al., 1982.)

subunits from the cDNAs and injected them into *Xenopus* oocytes. When all four RNAs were injected, functional ACh channels, which produced inward currents with applied acetylcholine and were blocked by tubocurarine, were expressed in the egg cell membrane. The injected RNA had instructed the protein synthetic mechanism in the egg cell to produce *Torpedo* ACh receptor channels! When less than four mRNAs were injected, poor responses or no responses to ACh were seen. Methfessel et al. (1986) used this method to express ACh channels and then studied them with the patch-clamp technique. The conductances and kinetic parameters of the channels were about the same as in living muscle membranes, indicating that the essential properties of the channels had been coded in the injected mRNAs. Scientists now could not only analyze the structure of channels, they could manufacture ribonucleic acids that would grow the channels in living cell membranes.

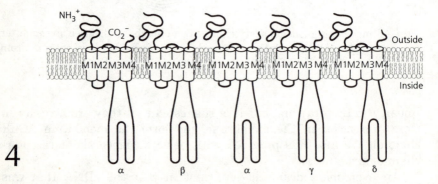

4

Theoretical assembly of four types of subunits in the membrane to form an ACh receptor (suggested by Mishina et al., 1984).

SODIUM CHANNELS

The history of biochemical studies of the sodium channel parallels that of the acetylcholine receptor strongly, for one main reason: There exists, for the sodium channel as well as for the acetylcholine receptor, a class of neurotoxins that bind covalently to the channel proteins and that can be used to separate them from membrane homogenates. In sodium channel studies tetrodotoxin or saxitoxin was radiolabeled and attached to a sepharose column to extract the channel molecules. The major component in the Na^+ channel proteins from electroplax was a large peptide of molecular weight 260 kDa (Agnew et al., 1980). The sodium channel in rat brain homogenates, on the other hand, had three main components, α, β_1, and β_2, with molecular weights of 260, 39, and 37 kDa (Messner and Catterall, 1985). All three components were heavily glycosylated, that is, they contained complex carbohydrate chains.

When the purified brain Na^+ channel protein was incorporated into lipid bilayers (Hartshorne et al., 1985), it was possible to resolve single-channel currents such as those in Figure 5. The percentage of time during which the channels were open increased with increasingly positive membrane potentials. Tetrodotoxin reversibly blocked the current through the channels. The P_K/P_{Na} ratio was about 0.14, compared to 0.07 for native channels, and the single-channel conductance with 0.5 M salt concentrations was 25 pS. Thus, with respect to voltage sensitivity, TTX block, and selectivity, the purified proteins had the same properties as native Na^+ channels.

PRIMARY STRUCTURE OF SODIUM CHANNELS

The structure of the α subunit was worked out in the same way as that of the acetylcholine receptor (Noda et al., 1984). By cloning and sequence analysis of cDNA for the electroplax Na^+ channel, Noda and co-workers determined that the protein consisted of 1,820 amino acids, arranged in a known order. Four REPEATED HOMOLOGY UNITS were also identified in the protein, with many amino acids in the same relative positions. The homologous domains each contained six membrane-spanning segments, as deduced from a hydrophilicity profile like that of Figure 3. This arrangement is shown in Figure 6. The Na^+ channel is formed by apposition of the four domains, with negatively charged residues exposed on the lumenal side. While the AChR channel consists of five peptides of four segments each, the Na^+ channel uses a single peptide with four homologous domains.

Some speculations about the voltage-sensing mechanism in sodium

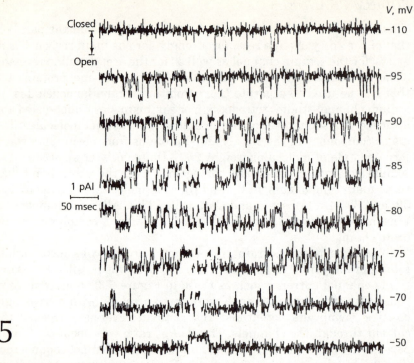

Currents recorded from reconstituted Na⁺ channels in lipid bilayer. Channels extracted from rat brain with bound saxitoxin in column, then incorporated into bilayers. (From Hartshorne et al., 1985.)

channels have also come from these molecular studies. Noda et al. (1984) suggested that, since the S4 segments in each domain are positively charged, they might serve as the voltage-sensing gates for the sodium channels. Measurement of gating currents has suggested that six electronic charges must cross the membrane to cause a single channel opening (Chapter 7). Since the S4 segments have an α-helical structure, it has been proposed that voltage-sensing might consist of a partial translocation of the segments, removing negative charges from the outside of the membrane and adding them to the inside (Catterall, 1986; Guy and Seetharamulu, (1986). This is known as the *sliding helix model.*

POTASSIUM CHANNELS

The determination of the structure of K⁺ channels was done differently from studies of Na⁺ and ACh channel structures. Because no known specific neurotoxin or other agent binds irreversibly to these channels, none can be used to purify them from membrane homogenates. Instead, a genetic analysis has been performed on *Drosophila* mutants that shake when exposed to ether; the mutant gene is thus called *Shaker*. Studies with mutants have shown that this gene encodes a component of the potassium channels carrying transient outward or A currents in these membranes (Salkoff and Wyman, 1981; Wu and Haugland, 1985; Timpe and Jan, 1987).

In 1987, Papazian et al., Kamb et al., and Baumann et al. succeeded in mapping the region of the altered genes in mutant flies and cloning cDNAs from the region. Tempel et al. (1987) then published the nucleotide sequences of two of these cDNA clones. From an analysis of the hydrophobicity profiles (like that of Figure 3), they concluded that the predicted peptide had several membrane-spanning segments and a region homologous to the S4 segment in the sodium channel. The molecular weight of the *Shaker* protein is only about 70 kDa, compared to 260 kDa for the sodium channel. Thus, an unknown number of copies of the structure (perhaps four) may assemble to form channels (Figure 7). The presence of the S4-like segment in the peptide led Tempel et al. (1987) to predict that the *Shaker* region would express an ion channel in a living membrane.

Timpe and co-workers (1988) and Iverson et al. (1988) were not long in testing this prediction. They made mRNAs from the cDNA clones with RNA polymerase and injected the mRNAs into *Xenopus* oocytes. The result was an inactivating outward (A-type) current such as that shown in Figure 8. The reversal potential of the tail currents

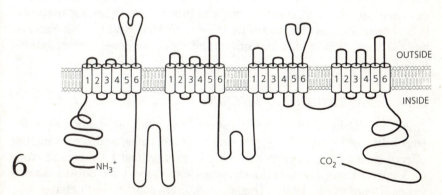

6

Molecular model of sodium channel. Four repeated homology domains, consisting of six segments each, occur within a single channel protein. Apposition of domains in the membrane forms the channel. (After Catterall, 1988.)

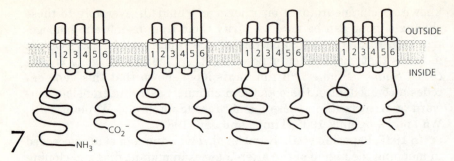

7

Structure of *Shaker* potassium channel inferred from sequencing of cDNA. Identical membrane-spanning subunits thought to associate to form a single channel. (After Tempel et al., 1987.)

varied with external [K] almost like the Nernst relation, the range of activation potentials was the same as the A-current in the insect muscle, and the oocyte current was blocked by 4-aminopyridine. In essence, the cloned cDNA had encoded an A-type potassium channel.

Another interesting result of the genetic analysis of K^+ currents is the discovery that genes similar to that for the A-current channels also code for delayed, or K^+ currents (Tempel et al., 1988; Wei et al., 1990). This may be explained by alternative splicing of the *Shaker* gene, producing products with greater or lesser degrees of homology, which in turn carry currents that activate more or less slowly, and do or do not inactivate. It may turn out that all potassium channels are made by different subfamilies of the same highly homologous gene family. Instead of drawing comparisons between different types of outward currents and classifying them into A or K types, for instance, it is now more useful to examine their diversity (Rudy, 1988; Serrano and Getting, 1989), with an understanding of the genetic mechanisms leading to it.

SITE-DIRECTED MUTAGENESIS

Another benefit of the genetic approach to channel structures is the possibility of intentionally altering channel genes and observing the effects on membrane currents. This is exemplified by a recent study of A-current inactivation in channels expressed by modified *Shaker* genes (Hoshi et al., 1990). These researchers constructed deletion mutants by chopping off more or less of the *N*-terminal ends of *Shaker*

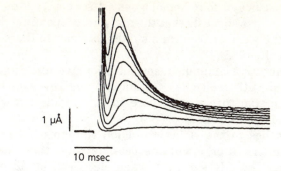

8

1 μÅ

10 msec

Expression of A currents in oocyte membrane by RNA prepared from *Shaker* cDNA. (From Timpe et al., 1988.)

cDNAs and injecting the fragments into *Xenopus* oocytes. All the mutants with deletions up to the first 22 amino acids showed smaller rates of entering the inactivated state and greater rates of return from inactivation (slowed or blocked inactivation). All of the mutations that caused deletions above amino acid 22 left inactivation intact. These results suggested that the first 22 amino acids near the amino end of the molecule form a domain that is important to inactivation. This study shows the power of the directed-mutation approach to yield detailed information about the role of specific parts of channel structures in processes of excitation.

OTHER CHANNEL STRUCTURES

Many other types of channels have been studied by similar methods of molecular biochemistry. Among the transmitter-activated channels, gamma-aminobutyric acid (GABA) channels have been isolated and purified (Siegel and Barnard, 1984; Marmalaki et al., 1987), as have glycine receptor channels (Graham et al., 1985). Like the ACh receptor, the subunits of these channels have been cloned and expressed in oocytes (Schofield et al., 1987; Levitan et al., 1988). The amino acid sequences have a high degree of homology with the ACh receptor, indicating that they may all come from a similar genetic origin.

The best-studied voltage-activated channel besides the Na^+ channel is the Ca^{2+} channel. This channel has been isolated from muscle membranes and the cDNA has been cloned and sequenced (Tanabe et al., 1987). A high degree of homology with the Na^+ channel was found, including the presence of four homologous S4 segments. Analysis of hydrophobicity profiles suggests that the membrane-spanning portions of the Ca^{2+} channels are arrayed in a similar manner to those of Na^+ channels (Catterall, 1988).

The nonregenerative channels responsible for GAP JUNCTIONS have also been studied with molecular techniques and revealed to be a double-hexameric structure with a pore in the middle (Unwin and Zampighi, 1980; Nicholson et al., 1983).

These approaches to the structure of ion channels have yielded much valuable information about the possible ways that molecules could move under the effect of membrane electric fields to perform their functions of signaling, contraction, secretion, etc. As more detailed knowledge comes in, the need will increase for synthetic modeling of membrane processes in order to discover whether individual mechanisms can work together to give accurate predictions of cell behavior.

PROBLEMS

1. If the density of sodium channels in the squid axon is $553/\mu m^2$, what is the spacing between the channels in angstroms if they are assumed to lie in a square array?

2. A phospholipid head group in a membrane occupies about 50 $Å^2$. Assuming there are 553 sodium channels per square micrometer and the rest of the membrane is phospholipid, what is the ratio of phospholipids to channels?

3. The voltage-sensitive block of sodium channels by quaternary local anesthetics (QX) is shown by applying different conditioning potentials, E_1 and E_2, in the presence of QX, and comparing the inward currents at some test potential at which the inward current is activated, such as 0 mV. If the first conditioning potential, E_1, is more positive than E_2, then more Na^+ channels will be open before the test potential is applied and the anesthetic block will be greater. If the second conditioning potential E_2 is −75 mV (where no Na^+ channels are open), and the first conditioning potential E_1 varies from −75 to +75 mV, draw a rough curve of $I(E_1)/I(E_2)$, the ratio of measured test currents as a function of conditioning potential.

4. Plot Equation 6 when E_2 varies from −75 to +75 mV in 0.5-mV steps, where

$$K_o = 210$$
$$[QX] = 0.5 \text{ m}M$$
$$E_2 = -75 \text{ mV}$$
$$\delta = 0.5$$

(For comparison, see Strichartz, 1973.)

5. What is the total molecular weight of the acetylcholine receptor channel, including all of the subunits?

6. What is the total molecular weight of the sodium channel from brain homogenates, including all of the subunits?

7. What would the weight of the *Shaker* potassium channel be if it were a homomultimer consisting of four identical subunits?

REFERENCES

Agnew, W. S., Moore, A. C., Levinson, S. R. and Raftery, M. A. 1980. Identification of a large molecular weight peptide associated with a tetrodotoxin binding protein from the electroplax of *Electrophorus electricus*. *Biochem. Biophys. Res. Commun.* 92, 860–866.

Armstrong, C. M. and Bezanilla, F. 1973. Currents related to movement of the gating particles of the sodium channels. *Nature (Lond.)* 242, 459–461.

Armstrong, C. M. and Hille, B. 1972. The inner quaternary ammonium ion receptor in potassium channels of the node of Ranvier. *J. Gen. Physiol.* 59, 388–400.

Baumann, A., Krah-Jentgens, I., Müller-Holtkamp, F., Seidel, R., Kecskemethy, N., Casal, J., Ferrus, A. and Pongs, O. 1987. Molecular organization of the maternal effect region of the *Shaker* complex of *Drosophila*: Characterization of an I_A channel transcript with homology to vertebrate Na^+ channel. *EMBO J.* 6, 3419–3429.

Catterall, W. A. 1986. Molecular properties of voltage-sensitive sodium channels. *Annu. Rev. Biochem.* 55, 953–985.

Catterall, W. A. 1988. Structure and function of voltage-sensitive ion channels. *Science* 242, 50–61.

Dwyer, T. M., Adams, D. J. and Hille, B. 1980. The permeability of the endplate channel to organic cations in frog muscle. *J. Gen. Physiol.* 75, 469–492.

Eaton, D. C., Brodwick, M. S., Oxford, G. S. and Rudy, B. 1978. Arginine-specific reagents remove sodium channel inactivation. *Nature (Lond.)* 271, 473–476.

Graham, D., Pfeiffer, F., Simler, R. and Betz, H. 1985. Purification and characterization of the glycine receptor of pig spinal cord. *Biochemistry* 24, 990–994.

Guy, H. R. and Seetharamulu, P. 1986. Molecular model of the action potential sodium channel. *Proc. Natl. Acad. Sci. USA* 83, 508–512.

Hartshorne, R. P., Keller, B. U., Talvenheimo, J. A., Catterall, W. A. and Montal, M. 1985. Functional reconstitution of the purified brain sodium channel in planar lipid bilayers. *Proc. Natl. Acad. Sci USA* 82, 240–244.

Hille, B. 1970. Ionic channels in nerve membranes. *Prog. Biophys. Mol. Biol.* 21, 1–32.

Hille, B. 1971. The permeability of the sodium channel to organic cations in myelinated nerve. *J. Gen. Physiol.* 58, 599–619.

Hille, B. 1972. The permeability of the sodium channel to metal cations in myelinated nerve. *J. Gen. Physiol.* 59, 637–658.

Hille, B. 1973. Potassium channels in myelinated nerve. Selective permeability to small cations. *J. Gen. Physiol.* 61, 669–686.

Hille, B. 1975a. Ionic selectivity of Na and K channels of nerve membranes. *Membranes- A Series of Advances, V. 3. : Lipid Bilayers and Biological Membranes: Dynamic Properties.* G. Eisenman (ed.). New York, Dekker, 255–323.

Hille, B. 1975b. Ionic selectivity, saturation and block in sodium channels. *J. Gen. Physiol.* 66, 535–560.

Hodgkin, A. L. and Huxley, A. F. 1952. A quantitative description of membrane current and its application to conduction and excitation in nerve. *J. Physiol.* 117, 500–544.

Hoshi, T., Zagotta, W. N. and Aldrich, R. W. 1990. Biophysical and molecular mechanisms of *Shaker* potassium channel inactivation. *Science* 250, 533–538.

Iverson, L. E., Tanouye, M. A., Lester, H. A., Davidson, N. and Rudy, B. 1988. A-type potassium channels expressed from *Shaker* locus cDNA. *Proc. Natl. Acad. Sci. USA* 85, 5723–5727.

Kamb, A., Iverson, L. E. and Tanouye, M. A. 1987. Molecular characterization of *Shaker*, a *Drosophila* gene that encodes a potassium channel. *Cell* 50, 405–413.

Karlsson, E., Heilbronn, E. and Widlund, L. 1972. Isolation of the nicotinic acetylcholine receptor by biospecific chromatography on insolubilized *Naja naja* neurotoxin. *FEBS Lett.* 28, 107–111.

Kistler, J., Stroud, R. M., Klymkowsky, M. W., Lalancette, R. A. and Fairclough, R. H. 1982. Structure and function of an acetylcholine receptor. *Biophys. J.* 37, 371–383.

Klymkowsky, M. W. and Stroud, R. M. 1979. Immunospecific identification and three-dimensional structure of a membrane-bound acetylcholine receptor from *Torpedo californica*. *J. Mol. Biol.* 128, 319–334.

Levitan, E. S., Blair, L. A. C., Dionne, V. E. and Barnard, E. A. 1988. Biophysical and pharmacological properties of cloned GABA$_A$ receptor subunits expressed in *Xenopus* oocytes. *Neuron* 1, 773–781.

Lindstrom, J., Anholt, R., Einarson, B., Engel, A., Osame, M. and Montal, M. 1980. Purification of acetylcholine receptors, reconstitution into lipid vesicles, and study of agonist-induced cation channel regulation. *J. Biol Chem.* 255, 8340–8350.

Marmalaki, C., Stephenson, F. A. and Barnard, E. A. 1987. The GABA$_A$/benzodiazepine receptor is a heterotetramer of homologous α and β subunits. *EMBO J.* 6, 561–565.

Methfessel, C., Witzemann, V., Takahashi, T., Mishina, M., Numa, S. and Sakmann, B. 1986. Patch clamp measurements on *Xenopus laevis* oocytes: Currents through endogenous channels and implanted acetylcholine receptors and sodium channels. *Pflügers Arch. Gesamte Physiol. Munschen Tiere* 407, 577–588.

Messner, D. J. and Catterall, W. A. 1985. The sodium channel from rat brain: separation and characterization of subunits. *J. Biol. Chem.* 260, 10597–10604.

Mishina, M., Kurosaki, T., Tobimatsu, T., Morimoto, Y., Noda, M., Yamamoto, T., Terao, M., Lindstrom, J., Takahashi, T., Kuno, M. and Numa, S. 1984. Expression of functional acetylcholine receptor from cloned cDNAs. *Nature (Lond.)* 307, 604–608.

Nicholson, B. J., Takemoto, L. H., Hunkapiller, M. W., Hood, L. E. and Revel, J. P. 1983. Differences between liver gap junction protein and lens MIP26 from rat: implications for tissue specificity of gap junctions. *Cell* 32, 967–978.

Noda, M., Takahashi, H., Tanabe, T., Toyosato, M., Furutani, Y., Hirose, T., Asai, M., Inayama, S., Miyata, T. and Numa, S. 1982. Primary structure of α-subunit precursor of *Torpedo californica* acetylcholine receptor deduced from cDNA sequence. *Nature (Lond.)* 299, 793–797.

Noda, M., Takahashi, T., Tanabe, T., Toyosato, M., Kikyotani, S., Hirose, T., Asai, M., Takashima, H., Inayama, S., Miyata, T. and Numa, S. 1983a. Primary structures of β- and δ-subunit precursors of *Torpedo californica* acetylcholine receptor deduced from cDNA sequences. *Nature (Lond.)* 301, 251–255.

Noda, M., Takahashi, H., Tanabe, T., Toyosato, M., Kikyotani, S., Furutani, Y., Hirose, T., Takashima, H., Inayama, S., Miyata, T. and Numa, S. 1983b. Structural homology of *Torpedo californica* acetylcholine receptor subunits. *Nature (Lond.)* 302, 528–532.

Noda, M., Shimizu, S., Tanabe, T., Takai, T., Kayano, T., Ikeda, T., Takahashi, H., Nakayama, H., Kanaoka, Y., Minamino, N., Kangawa, K., Matsuo, H., Raftery, M. A., Hirose, T., Inayama, S., Hayashida, H., Miyata, T. and Numa, S. 1984. Primary structure of *Electrophorus electricus* sodium channel deduced from cDNA sequence. *Nature (Lond.)* 312, 121–127.

Papazian, D. M., Schwarz, T. L., Tempel, B. L., Jan, Y. N. and Jan, L. Y. 1987. Cloning of genomic and complememtary DNA from *Shaker*, a putative potassium channel gene from *Drosophila*. *Science* 237, 749–753.

Raftery, M. A. 1973. Isolation of acetylcholine receptor-α-bungarotoxin complexes from *Torpedo californica* electroplax. *Arch. Biochem. Biophys.* 154, 270–276.

Raftery, M. A., Hunkapiller, M. W., Strader, C. D. and Hood, L. E. 1980. Acetylcholine receptor: complex of homologous subunits. *Science* 208, 1454–1457

Ross, M. J., Klymkowsky, M. W., Agard, D. A. and Stroud, R. M. 1977. Structural studies of a membrane-bound acetylcholine receptor from *Torpedo californica*. *J. Mol. Bol.* 116, 635–659.

Rudy, B. 1988. Diversity and ubiquity of potassium channels. *Neuroscience* 25, 729–749.

Salkoff, L. and Wyman, R. 1981. Genetic modifications of potassium channels in *Drosophila Shaker* mutants. *Nature (Lond.)* 293, 228–230.

Schofield, P. R., Darlison, M. G., Fujita, N., Burt, D. R., Stephenson, F. A., Rodriguez, H., Rhee, L. M., Ramachandran, J., Reale, V., Glencourse, T. A., Seeburg, P. G. and Barnard, E. A. 1987. Sequence and functional expression of the $GABA_A$ receptor shows a ligand-gated receptor super-family. *Nature (Lond.)* 328, 221–227.

Serrano, E. E. and Getting, P. A. 1989. Diversity of the transient outward potassium current in somata of identified molluscan neurons. *J. Neurosci.* 9, 4021–4032.

Siegel, E. and Barnard, E. A. 1984. A γ-aminobutyric/benzodiazepine receptor complex from bovine cerebral cortex. *J. Biol. Chem.* 259, 7219–7223.

Strichartz, G. R. 1973. The inhibition of sodium currents in myelinated nerve by quaternary derivatives of lidocaine. *J. Gen. Physiol.* 62, 37–57.

Tanabe, T., Takashima, H., Mikami, A., Flockerzi, V., Takahashi, H., Kangawa, K., Kojima, M., Matsuo, H., Hirose, T. and Numa, S. 1987. Primary structure of the receptor for calcium channel blockers from skeletal muscle. *Nature (Lond.)* 328, 313–318.

Tempel, B. L., Papazian, D. M., Schwarz, T. L., Jan, Y. N. and Jan, L. Y. 1987. Sequence of a probable potassium channel component encoded at *Shaker* locus of *Drosophila*. *Science* 237, 770–775.

Tempel, B. L., Jan, Y. N. and Jan, L. Y. 1988. Cloning of a probable potassium channel gene from mouse brain. *Nature (Lond.)* 332, 837–839.

Timpe, L. C. and Jan, L. Y. 1987. Gene dosage and complementation analysis of the *Shaker* locus in *Drosophila*. *J. Neurosci.* 7, 1307–1317.

Timpe, L. C., Schwarz, T. L., Tempel, B. L., Papazian, D. M., Jan, Y. N. and Jan, L. Y. 1988. Expression of functional potassium channels from *Shaker* cDNA in *Xenopus* oocytes. *Nature (Lond.)* 331, 143–145.

Unwin, P. N. T. and Zampighi, G. 1980. Structure of the junction between communicating cells. *Nature (Lond.)* 283, 545–549.

Wei, A., Covarrubias, M., Butler, A., Baker, K., Pak, M. and Salkoff, L. 1990. K^+ current diversity is produced by an extended gene family conserved in *Drosophila* and mouse. *Science* 248, 599–603.

Woodhull, A. 1973. Ionic blockage of sodium channels in nerve. *J. Gen. Physiol.* 61, 687–708.

Wu, C.-F. and Haugland, F. N. 1985. Voltage clamp analysis of membrane currents in larval muscle fibers of *Drosophila*: alteration of potassium currents in *Shaker* mutants. *J. Neurosci.* 5, 2626–2640.

Wu, W. C.-S., Moore, H.-P. H and Raftery, M. A. 1981. Quantitation of cation transport by reconstituted membrane vesicles containing purified acetylcholine receptor. *Proc. Natl. Acad. Sci. USA* 78, 775–779.

14

NEW DIRECTIONS

This has been a brief exposure to cellular neurophysiology and many of its current theories. Such a presentation cannot be complete, due to the recent explosion of information about the nervous system. The subjects of nerve and muscle development, neuroendocrinology, immunology, and axoplasmic transport have perforce been largely omitted, although doubtless many valuable contributions will come from these and other areas. In this chapter some challenging new approaches to the study of excitable membranes will be described, and an attempt made to place this subject in a context for studying the nervous system in general.

NEUROMODULATION

This is a general heading for studies dealing with alterations of membrane electrical properties in response to hormonal or synaptic stimulation. It has developed from an awareness of the importance of intracellular SECOND MESSENGERS such as cyclic adenosine monophosphate (cAMP) and inositol trisphosphate (IP3) in regulating ion channel activity. This approach has led to some significant advances in our understanding of how cell membrane potentials and conductances are controlled by neurotransmitters, especially on a larger time scale.

Figure 1 is a general scheme of the function of second messengers. When the transmitter (T) binds to the receptor (R), a membrane-bound hydrolytic enzyme (MBE) is activated (in some cases by a guanosine triphosphate binding protein; Rodbell, 1980; Gilman, 1984) and catalyzes the production of a second messenger molecule. Second messen-

244

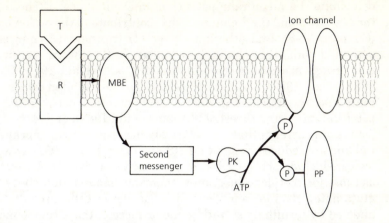

Role of intracellular second messengers in neuromodulation. T, transmitter; R, receptor; MBE, membrane bound enzyme; PK, protein kinase; P, high-energy phosphate; PP, phosphoprotein. Further details in the text.

gers include cyclic AMP, inositol trisphosphate, and diacylglycerol. The second messenger may activate a protein kinase (PK) or act directly on some other intracellular system. The protein kinases catalyze hydrolysis of ATP and phosphorylation of membrane ion channels or intracellular phosphoproteins (PP).

Cyclic AMP is produced by hydrolysis of ATP by a membrane-bound adenylate cyclase. It is thought to play a role in β-adrenergic transmission (where norepinephrine acts as the transmitter); in the modulation of bursting in molluscan neurons (Adams and Benson, 1985); and in various potassium currents in molluscan and vertebrate neurons (Kaczmarek and Levitan, 1987). Inositol trisphosphate is produced by cleavage of phosphatidyl inositol by a membrane phosphodiesterase when triggered by receptor activation. IP3 then diffuses in the cytoplasm and releases Ca^{2+} from intracellular stores (Fink et al., 1988). Systems such as this affect a variety of membrane conductances that are sensitive to externally applied neurotransmitters (Kaczmarek and Levitan, 1987). They are likely to determine the membrane potentials of cells on long time scales, such as diurnal rhythms, and may contribute to long-term potentiation of synaptic responses (Koyano et al., 1985).

ION-CHANNEL DIVERSITY

Along with the above types of channels that are affected by intracellular second messengers, a plethora of other channel types normally determine the membrane potentials in excitable cells. These include the Na^+, K^+, and Ca^{2+} channels that contribute to the action potential (Chapters 5–8), and others such as: (1) transient (A) and calcium-activated potassium channels (Chapter 7); (2) inward rectifier channels (Hagiwara and Takahashi, 1974; Ciani et al., 1978; Constanti and Galvan, 1983); (3) M-currents, muscarine-inhibited potassium currents that are activated in the range of potentials between the resting potential and firing threshold (Adams et al., 1982); and (4) S-currents, potassium currents that are relatively insensitive to membrane potential and are reduced by serotonin (Siegelbaum et al., 1982). In addition, we can include the long list of transmitter-activated channels, such as those for acetylcholine, norepinephrine, gamma-aminobutyric acid, glutamate, glycine, and dopamine, as nerve cells are likely to be affected by terminals secreting one or more of these compounds.

The electrical properties of different types of nerve cells are a result of the particular channels present in the cell membranes; these determine, for instance, whether a cell is normally silent or active, or whether it discharges regularly or in bursts. From studies of channel structure, it appears that single channel types or channel families may be determined by single genes or gene families (Stevens, 1987; Wei et al., 1990). This implies that cells may alter their electrical properties simply by the types of channels they synthesize. This powerful idea has redirected the emphasis of researchers from analyzing one type of current or channel to placing each channel in a genetic taxonomy (Schauf, 1987; Rudy, 1988; Serrano and Getting, 1989). One interesting result from studies of this kind is that many of the known voltage-activated structures have a common property: They contain the S4 segment found in the sodium channel. This presumed voltage-sensing segment may have been conserved in evolution from ancient Ca^{2+}-channels (Hille, 1992).

Studying ion channels with the patch-clamp technique may give the impression that action potentials and synaptic potentials are kinds of epiphenomena and not central to the function of excitable cells. However, it should be remembered that it is the changing membrane potential during the spike that causes propagation, both in the axon and sarcolemma. This results from *summed* channel currents that are only large enough to produce a threshold depolarization on a macroscopic scale. Postsynaptic potentials only sum to produce excitation in a millivolt range, where currents are in microamperes rather than picoamperes. Functions such as propagation, summation, and threshold detection do not occur on a single-channel level; the currents are too small. This leads to a final comment on levels of study of excitable systems.

DIVERSITY IN RESEARCH

The preface to this volume points out the trend toward reductionism that has occurred over the years in studies of brain and nerve functions. This may be inevitable in the development of a field; it certainly occurred in physics in the 1930s, when splitting of spectroscopic lines became fine and then hyperfine, as new atomic orbitals were described. This research led to the development of the atomic theory, the uncertainty principle, and quantum electrodynamics, among other systems of analysis. Likewise, in excitable membrane biophysics, with each reduction of the level of experimental subject matter we have gained a new degree of understanding. Reduction is an effective means of explaining previously studied higher levels of behavior, at least in part. However, the fact that one aspect of a higher function has been explained does not mean that level is completely understood. Knowing that ion channels produce action potentials, for instance, does not tell us all the possible types of action potentials, nor how the spike width varies with repetition, nor how spike discharges occur in bursts, nor how the timing of action potentials functions in networks of neurons.

Figure 2 is a schematic representation of some of the possible levels of study of nervous structures. While not inclusive, it indicates the types of studies that may be, and are, carried out at each level of detail. Different methods of structural observations with optical or electronic methods are also suggested for several levels of investigation. The point is that each level still contains undiscovered realms of useful information. While we may, in fact, know which gene determines which type of ion channel in the near future, it is unlikely that this information will completely describe even a single nerve network, since networks embody specific anatomical and physiological properties. To carry the analogy further, it is indeed difficult to argue that an understanding of the properties of every known type of nerve cell in the brain would shed a glimmer of light on psychological measures such as preference and avoidance. For this reason, diversity in research should not only be encouraged, but it seems a prerequisite to further progress at each level of inquiry.

REFERENCES

Adams, P. R., Brown, D. A. and Constanti, A. 1982. M-currents and other potassium currents in bullfrog sympathetic neurones. *J. Physiol.* 330, 537–572.

Adams, W. B. and Benson, J. A. 1985. The generation and modulation of endogenous rhythmicity in the *Aplysia* bursting pacemaker neurone R15. *Prog. Biophys. Mol. Biol.* 46, 1–49.

Atomic–Molecular Theories
Chemical bond theory
Reaction energies
Diffusion potentials

Membrane Structures
Lipid and protein biochemistry
Genetic determination
X-ray diffraction

Single Ion Channels
Voltage and ligand sensitivity
Stochastic properties
Electron microscopy

Electrical Phenomena in Cells
Resting and action potential
Synaptic transmission
Neuronal development

Complex Behavior of Cells
Repetitive firing, bursting
Facilitation, depression
Intracellular dyes

Patterned Interaction of Cells
Central pattern generators
Nerve networks
Light microscopy

CNS functions
Detection and recognition
Integration and coordination
Anatomy

Organism Behavior
Learning and memory
Decision making
Movement

Complex Social Behavior
Cooperation and hostility
Motivation
Language

2

Levels of investigation of nervous structures, including the brain, with examples of techniques used for each level. Most detailed at top, becoming increasingly more complex. Methods of visualization of structures indicated at the bottom of some levels.

Ciani, S., Krasne, S., Miyazaki, S. and Hagiwara, S. 1978. A model for anomalous rectification: Electrochemical-potential-dependent gating of membrane channels. *J. Membr. Biol.* 44, 103–134.

Constanti, A. and Galvan, M. 1983. Fast inward-rectifying current accounts for anomalous rectification in olfactory cortex neurons. *J. Physiol.* 335, 153–178.

Fink, L. A., Connor, J. A. and Kaczmarek, L. K. 1988. Inositol trisphosphate releases intracellularly stored calcium and modulates ion channels in molluscan neurons. *J. Neurosci.* 8, 2544–2555.

Gilman, A. G. 1984. G proteins and dual control of adenylate cyclase. *Cell* 36, 577–579.

Hagiwara, S. and Takahashi, K. 1974. The anomalous rectification and cation selectivity of the membrane of a starfish egg cell. *J. Membr. Biol.* 18, 61–80.

Hille, B. 1992. *Ionic Channels of Excitable Membranes*, Second Edition. Sunderland, Mass., Sinauer.

Kaczmarek, L. K. and Levitan, I. B. 1987. *Neuromodulation: The Biochemical Control of Neuronal Excitability*. New York, Oxford.

Koyano, K., Kuba, K. and Minota, S. 1985. Long-term potentiation of transmitter release induced by repetitive presynaptic activities in bullfrog sympathetic ganglia. *J. Physiol.* 359, 219–233.

Rodbell, M. 1980. The role of hormone receptors and GTP-regulatory proteins in membrane transduction, *Nature (Lond.)* 284, 17–22.

Rudy, B. 1988. Diversity and ubiquity of K channels. *Neuroscience* 25, 729–749.

Schauf, C. L. 1987. Ion channel diversity: A revolution in biology? *Sci. Prog. (Oxford)* 71, 459–478.

Serrano, E. E. and Getting, P. A. 1989. Diversity of the transient outward potassium current in somata of identified molluscan neurons. *J. Neurosci.* 9, 4021–4032.

Siegelbaum, S. A., Camardo, J. S. and Kandel, E. R. 1982. Serotonin and cyclic AMP close single K^+ channels in *Aplysia* sensory neurones. *Nature (Lond.)* 299, 413–417.

Stevens, C. F. 1987. Channel families in the brain. *Nature (Lond.)* 328, 198–199.

Wei, A., Covarrubias, M., Butler, A., Baker, K., Pak, M. and Salkoff, L. 1990. K^+ current diversity is produced by an extended gene family conserved in *Drosophila* and mouse. *Science* 248, 599-603.

SOLUTIONS TO CHAPTER-END PROBLEMS

CHAPTER 1

1. α: 33 m/sec; β: 21 m/sec

2. Fast peak: 98 m/sec;
   slow peak: 19 m/sec

3. 9.3 m/sec/μm

4. 3.3 cm

5. 100 kΩ

CHAPTER 2

1. 3.0

2. $R = 728$ kΩ; $C = 0.170$ μF

3. $R_m = 3660$ $\Omega\cdot$cm^2;
   $C_m = 33.9$ μF/cm^2

4. 0.124 sec

5. 33.9

6. 0.124 M$\Omega\cdot$cm^2

7. 1.93

8. 9.5×10^{-4} cm; 0.308

CHAPTER 3

1. -75.3 mV

2. 54.6 mV; -66.3 mV

3. -48.9 mV

4. -36.5 mV

5. 235 mM

6. 235 mM

7. 0.028

8. Sequence 2

9. -48.9 mV

10. -38.6 mV

11. $I = \dfrac{2Fk_i u_2 [\text{K}]_o}{k_o} \sinh(EF/2RT)$

CHAPTER 4

1. -215 mV

2. -88.2 mV

3. -91.9 mV

4. $E = \dfrac{rg_K E_K + g_{Na} E_{Na}}{rg_K + g_{Na}}$

5. -88.2 mV

6. -92.4 mV

7. -35.6 mV

8. -48.9 mV

9. 761/μm^2

10. 6.064

CHAPTER 5

1. $+50$ mV

4. Peak $g_{Na} = 13.3$ mS/cm^2;
   final $g_K = 22.7$ mS/cm^2

CHAPTER 6

1. 15.2 mS/cm^2

2. 13.4 mS/cm^2

4. 10^{-7} coulomb/cm^2

5. 1.04 pmol/cm^2

6. 45.5

CHAPTER 7

1. 15.1 mS/cm^2

2. 9.64×10^{12}

3. 13.8/μm^2

4. 2867/μm^2

5. 5.23 to 7.00 pS

CHAPTER 8

1. 29 mV
2. 8.73 mV
4. −75.4 mV
5. 33 mV
6. 0.3 nM

CHAPTER 9

3. $I = \dfrac{A/t + B}{R_m(1 - e^{-t/\tau_m})}$

CHAPTER 10

1. 0.566
2. 186
3. 30
4. 6304
5. $3.61 \times 10^{-7}\ M$
6. 68.2 mV
7. 2200

CHAPTER 11

4. 2.34 pA
5. 1.46×10^7 ions/sec
6. 10,220 ions/channel
7. 4.3 channels/μm^2

CHAPTER 12

1. 23.5 pS
2. 32.0 pS
3. 38.5 msec
4. 40.0 msec
5. $p_{C_1} + p_{C_2} + p_O = 1$
6. State O
7. $I_K = \overline{g_K} P_O (E - E_K)$

CHAPTER 13

1. 423 Å
2. 3617:1
5. 255 kDa
6. 336 kDa
7. 280 kDa

ILLUSTRATION CREDITS

Page 37: Courtesy of the Physiological Society.

Page 67: From *Journal of General Physiology* 94:511. Copyright 1989 Rockefeller University Press.

Page 73: Courtesy of the Ciba Foundation.

Page 104: Reprinted by permission of Charles C. Thomas, Publishers.

Page 119: Reprinted by permission of Raven Press.

Page 125: Reprinted by permission of Pergamon Press.

Page 162: Courtesy of the Physiological Society.

Page 180: Figure 7: Courtesy of the Physiological Society.

Page 200: Reprinted by permission of Pergamon Press.

Page 205: From *Nature* 285:140. Copyright 1980, Macmillan Magazines Ltd.

Page 206: From *Nature* 287:447. Copyright 1980, Macmillan Magazines Ltd.

Page 207: From *Nature* 282:863. Copyright 1979, Macmillan Magazines Ltd.

Page 224: From *Journal of General Physiology* 79:333. Copyright 1982 Rockefeller University Press.

Page 230: From *Journal of General Physiology* 66:535. Copyright 1975 Rockefeller University Press.

Page 233: Drawing by Robert M. Stroud, University of California/San Francisco.

Page 234: Figure 3: From *Nature* 299:733. Copyright 1982, Macmillan Magazines Ltd.

Page 237: From *Science* 242:50. Copyright 1988 by the American Association for the Advancement of Science.

Page 238: From *Science* 237:770. Copyright 1987 by the American Association for the Advancement of Science.

Page 239: From *Nature* 331:143. Copyright 1988, Macmillan Magazines Ltd.

INDEX